Love & Peace,

Cathlin Duncan

Praise for Everyday Awakening

"In this beautifully written, intelligent, yet heart-centered work, Catherine Duncan has merged a traditional religious orientation with cutting-edge psychological insights and tools that will empower the aspiring soul on its way to awakening."

JOHN RUSKAN

author of *Emotional Clearing* and *Deep Clearing*

"While many traditional religions focus on being 'chosen,' spirituality is, in the end, about what we choose. In *Everyday Awakening*, Catherine Duncan reminds us that awakening isn't an incident—it's an action, one we're each capable of taking. Duncan, who's been through some harrowing experiences herself, serves as a loving guide on the path to awakening as a way of life."

TERRI TRESPICIO

author of *Unfollow Your Passion: How to Create a Life That Matters to You*

"How to awaken? That is the question and Catherine Duncan has the answer. She draws on her decades of spiritual practice and her deep humanity to point you in the right direction and to instill your journey with purpose and meaning."

RICHARD J. LEIDER

bestselling author of *The Power of Purpose*, *Repacking Your Bags*, and *Who Do You Want to Be When You Grow Old?*

"I AM ALIVE. Can you embrace that statement and wear it boldly? Sense your soul in the poetry of every moment? You deserve to—and Catherine Duncan's book, *Everyday Awakening*, points the way to loving every darn second of your existence. This is more than another self-help assurance of 'happily ever after.' Catherine's gritty life experiences, including childhood cancer and serving as a hospice chaplain, means that every point made and practice shared is gripping and powerful. This is not just another self-help guidebook; it's an initiation into everyday and genuine enlightenment."

CYNDI DALE

author of 30-plus internationally renowned books about energy healing, including the award-winning *The Subtle Body* series and *Energy Healing for Trauma, Stress & Chronic Illness*

"The word 'breathe' in Japanese is written with two characters, 'heart' and 'self,' and the two together spell 'presence.' Catherine Duncan's new book is both a metaphor for and an embodiment of this great wisdom."

PETER M. LITCHFIELD, PHD

president, Professional School of Behavioral Health Sciences

"Catherine Duncan is an amazing catalyst for healing. Her work with the hundreds of patients I have referred to her is so beautiful that I can be moved to tears. If you are suffering in mind, body, or spirit, or if you feel stuck in negativity and want to move forward, then this book of wisdom will be worth more than its weight in gold. May you follow these five practices and be transformed."

GREG PLOTNIKOFF, MD, MTS, FACP

founder and medical director, Minnesota Personalized Medicine

"We yearn for authenticity as much as aliveness, and *Everyday Awakening* offers both. Catherine Duncan has clearly walked the paths she guides us on. Her five practices for awakening are practical and accessible yet profoundly soulful. Use them and breathe deep into your own vibrant life."

HENRY EMMONS, MD
author of *The Chemistry of Joy* and *The Chemistry of Calm*, cohost of the podcast *Joy Lab*

"Catherine Duncan's book will help you avoid becoming overwhelmed with anxiety and pain. Its five powerful practices will allow you to harness your psychology and, in turn, your life. This book will help you turn your suffering into an awakening and lead you to find inner peace."

MARK FORD
former chief revenue officer of Time Inc.

"*Everyday Awakening* is a beautiful guide to living a more vibrant, joy-filled life. Catherine Duncan teaches us what it means to live fully, drawing on her years of walking with people at the end of life. You'll feel Catherine's wisdom and radiant heart as you follow the five practices and awaken your heart and soul. This book has the power to transform our individual and collective lives."

SHAUNA SHAPIRO, PHD
professor, author of *Good Morning, I Love You: Mindfulness and Self-Compassion Practices to Rewire Your Brain for Calm, Clarity, and Joy*

"*Everyday Awakening* is your road map to living a fully engaged life. Catherine's story and her five practices are refreshingly accessible. She doesn't just talk about awakening—she's lived it, and teaches you how to stop sleepwalking through your life and start living it!"

MEL ROBBINS
New York Times bestselling author and host of *The Mel Robbins Podcast*

"If you are now standing at a crossroad, not knowing which path to take for your life journey—because of pain, anxiety, confusion, and suffering of all kinds—and looking for a guide and role model to lead you out of the woods, Catherine Duncan is the perfect one for you.

"In her book, through her own life experiences, she not only teaches you how to find your path. She also shows you how to choose a life that holds true meaning and purpose for you."

GRAND MASTER CHUNYI LIN
founder and creator of Spring Forest Qigong

"*Everyday Awakening* is a beautiful reminder of what matters: the important process of being human. If you need direction to the root of self-healing, this book is it!"

DAVE RAKEL, MD
author of *The Compassionate Connection*, editor of *Integrative Medicine*, and chair of the Department of Family Medicine and Community Health, University of Wisconsin School of Medicine and Public Health

EVERYDAY AWAKENING

*Five Practices for Living Fully, Feeling Deeply,
and Coming into Your Heart and Soul*

CATHERINE DUNCAN

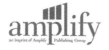

an imprint of Amplify Publishing Group

www.amplifypublishinggroup.com

Everyday Awakening: Five Practices for Living Fully,
Feeling Deeply, and Coming into Your Heart and Soul

For more information, please contact:
Amplify Publishing, an imprint of Amplify Publishing Group
620 Herndon Parkway, Suite 320
Herndon, VA 20170
info@amplifypublishing.com

Library of Congress Control Number: 2022923261

CPSIA Code: PRV0223A

ISBN-13: 978-1-63755-608-5

Printed in the United States

To my husband, Scott, who on our first date, at twenty-four years old, saw my path before I did. And to my children, Owen and Adria, for your inspiration and love.

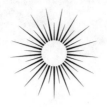

CONTENTS

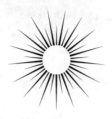

INTRODUCTION

What Does It Mean to Be Alive?

THE WAITING ROOM OF THE University of Minnesota hospital children's oncology clinic was packed. I looked around and saw other kids—kids with no hair, no arms, or no legs. I could hear more kids screaming and crying behind the doors of the medical rooms down the hallway. Terrified, I pretended to not be one of them as I adjusted the bandana over my wig. I looked down; I still had both of my legs. I purposely tried not to touch anything. By not touching anything, I could somehow feel like I wasn't part of this horror show.

The nurse called my name, and I walked into the grim medical room. I lay down on the hard table, and a doctor and nurses walked in, wearing white coats and carrying a tray with multiple large syringes. They gave me a peppermint to suck on as they started injecting chemotherapy agents into my arm. A chemical taste suddenly started running through my mouth. My mother stood next to me, holding my hand, and I could feel fear running through her body. There was not a sound in the room; everyone was staring at me.

As we left the hospital, my mother opened all the doors because I refused to touch anything.

At home, early evening, the nausea hit me. I went to my bedroom and started throwing up. It was the 1970s, and there were no anti-nausea drugs available. My mom slept next to me, holding my head every time I got sick.

I spent the next day on the couch, watching TV, as my mom was busy doing things around the house. All my older siblings were off to school. I felt weak, shaky, and full of fear. I didn't know if I could muster enough energy to get up to go to the bathroom.

No one was talking with me. My mother's love was comforting, but no one had said anything about what was really happening to me. I was walking on a tightrope between life and death. I could see over the cliff into the abyss.

I don't want to die.

The thought rushed through me. In that moment, I decided I wanted to live.

Out of nowhere, I started to pray: *Please, God, I want to live to be twenty years old.* I thought that if I lived to be twenty, I would see the world.

Until that moment, faith and God had meant nothing to me. My family attended a Lutheran church with some regularity, but we did not talk about faith or God—ever. There had been chaplains at the hospital, but no minister or counselor had come to speak with me while I was there.

I told no one of my prayers. I just kept praying. *Please, God, I want to live to be twenty years old.* I kept saying this prayer for days, maybe even weeks, as the chemotherapy and radiation appointments continued. *Please, God, I want to live to be twenty years old.*

One day, while I was praying, a feeling of peace and warmth suddenly flooded my body, followed by a pulsing aliveness. I felt a sense of something beyond come into me. Something not of this world was present with me.

I felt comforted. I was no longer alone. A knowing came to me: *I am okay.* I stopped questioning whether I was going to live or die; I *knew* I was going to live.

This childhood experience cracked me open. I was eleven years old. I'd been given only a 20 percent chance of surviving cancer. Yet I had lived. And I had awakened to the preciousness of being alive.

This first awakening experience set in motion my passion for understanding what it means to be fully alive. This passion followed me into adulthood. During my first career, in corporate advertising, I had a near-death experience, and afterward I quit my lucrative, successful job because my heart just wasn't in my work anymore. I changed direction and became a chaplain. Serving in a level-one trauma center and then in hospice, I walked with thousands of people as they navigated the rough terrain of upheaval, loss, and death. Many of them were searching for meaning as their lives were upended by trauma or a dire diagnosis. Again and again, I saw people who, facing their death as I had, felt the acute aliveness of just this moment. Walking with them, I learned even more about what awakening looks and feels like.

In 2016 I started my private practice as an integrative spiritual consultant so that I could help people who, like me, are seeking answers to the question of what it really means to be alive. Each of my clients comes from a different background and is facing their own unique circumstances, yet they have one thing in common:

all of them are experiencing a wake-up call, and it has started them on a search for more.

My client Jill, for example, was a leading doctor at a well-known medical center and had achieved and surpassed her career goals. But in her first Zoom meeting with me, she said, "I feel nothing. I feel dead."

She echoed the same sentiment another client, Rick, a longtime entrepreneur, had shared just that morning: "I have a great wife, two kids. I've achieved a lot, but I feel a gnawing inside. Something is missing."

Later in the afternoon, I saw Susan, a successful attorney for a large national law firm, who had pushed herself hard throughout her life and now, in her early fifties, had just been diagnosed with an autoimmune disease. "There has got to be more to life," she said. "I want to feel peace and ease."

The next morning I met Nate, who'd recently lost his wife. "I'm trying to make sense of my life. I need help," he told me.

Then I meet with Nicky, a woman in her midthirties who was a two-year Covid long-hauler and still dealing with challenging symptoms. She said, "I want to find balance and heal. I want to feel more."

Like the patients I saw when I was a chaplain, Susan, Nate, and Nicky were experiencing external wake-up calls. A painful loss; a difficult health condition; a sudden, unasked-for life change—these are just some of the external circumstances that can lead us to question whether more is possible for our lives. For others, like Jill and Rick, the call is an internal one. From the outside, it may look like they have it all, but inside they feel numb and empty. They feel like they're living on autopilot—going through the motions of life but not feeling like they're actually living it. They might even feel bored with life. Others in this situation may feel overstressed, anxious, depressed, or exhausted. Driven by their thoughts, which never seem to shut off, and by feelings of being less than or not enough, they often experience a constant pushing or striving, and they can find little rest and ease.

They are all on the cusp of *awakening*.

Whatever form their wake-up call takes, people who find their way to my practice usually have an innate sense that what they need is something in addition to and beyond standard physical and mental health care. That's where I come in: I work at the intersection of mental, physical, emotional, and spiritual health, which is exactly where awakening happens. Awakening is a whole-being experience. I blend my clinical knowledge of neuroscience and Western mental health care; my professional training in ministry, chaplaincy, and complementary healing modalities; and my personal experience living on the edge between life and death and learning what it means to be alive.

If you feel a desire for more, you are in the right place. My mission is to demystify awakening for you. In this book, I share five core practices that will allow you to awaken—to come into your heart and soul, live fully, and feel deeply—again and again in everyday moments.

In the first chapter, I will give you an overview of these five practices by sharing how I learned them. Unlike many people who have found them through spiritual traditions or teachers, I discovered them through raw, lived experience. I have been a student of these five awakening practices nearly my entire life and teaching them to others for the past twenty years. Today they are the five core practices I share with all my clients.

Chapters 2–6 will then explore each practice in depth. To illuminate the practices, I share stories of my own life; my family members and a few close friends have given me permission to include some of their experiences as well. In addition, I've included stories from current clients and patients I saw as a chaplain. The core of each client or patient's story is true and authentic; however, I have changed their names and specific identifying details to protect their privacy.

In each practice chapter, I provide a variety of exercises, including meditations, breath exercises, visualizations, movement, and sound-based exercises, and neuroscience-informed exercises. Using the ones that work best for you, you can experience the power of each practice for yourself and move from your thinking mind into your body, where we feel alive. This is how you step onto the path of awakening.

Awakening and each of the five practices are discussed in various spiritual and philosophical traditions, and modern science is showing us in more and more detail how our brains and other parts of our body are noticeably changed by these practices. Because my primary intention with this book is to help you practice awakening for yourself, I've chosen to focus on the how and why of it instead of taking you deep into the science behind it. I've also chosen not to explore how different traditions address awakening, for a couple of reasons. First, I firmly believe awakening is a universal human experience, and you don't need to follow a particular path or tradition to do it. Second, reading and learning about awakening may be inspiring for our minds, but it's not the same as experiencing and feeling awakening itself. If you are interested in learning more about awakening or any of the five practices through these lenses, I've provided lists of some of my favorite books in the "Additional Resources" section.

We all have the power to open, grow, and transform through

our lifetime. The more you choose to awaken—a lifelong journey for all of us—the more you can embody love, light, and peace and become a source of love and light in the world.

It is easy to live in a state of near slumber, unaware of being alive and the many blessings that are present for each of us daily. Either you're living on autopilot, or you're consciously choosing how you live each day.

What if today you chose to let your heart and your soul, instead of your mind, run your life?

What if you chose to embody more deep presence, love, and openness?

What if you chose to feel more ease, peace, and flow?

How do you want to live this precious life you've been given?

Do you want to feel fully alive?

You can choose to awaken right now.

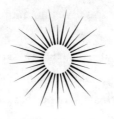

1

Five Practices for Awakening

AWAKENING IS A PROFOUND EXPERIENCE, but it is not mysterious or esoteric. It is not reserved for only a few rare mystics, holy saints, or "good people." Awakening is not just for followers of a few special spiritual traditions—or just for people who think of themselves as spiritual. Awakening is vital to our human spirit, and we are all naturally being pulled toward it.

Awakening is remembering our heart and soul and learning how to live more fully from them. When we are living from our heart and soul, rather than just our ego minds, we feel it physically, emotionally, and spiritually. It leads to a feeling of vibrant aliveness, a sharp sense of presence, and a tangible feeling of energy moving and flowing through us. I feel this aliveness as a vibration that courses through my body. It comes to me when I hear the enchanting calls of a flock of geese. I feel it when I stop in awe upon seeing the full moon light up the sky, illuminating the lake near my house, or when a friend or stranger greets me with a warm hello. It is a feeling of wonderment, warmth, and love and a knowing that says, "I am here, alive, right now!"

This aliveness culminates in a visceral sense of love and oneness with all of life. When we feel this oneness—whatever we may call it—the world opens up. Instead of our ego minds running our lives, we live aligned with our souls and this oneness. We are open to the fullness of life. Our lives are forever changed.

Awakening is often portrayed as something that happens to us, usually suddenly and spontaneously, and usually only once. But in fact, awakening is an action—an ongoing activity. It doesn't require traveling to a distant country or sitting at the feet of an enlightened guru or spiritual teacher. Though some people, including me, start their path of awakening during dramatic, life-or-death situations, anyone can start awakening right now, right where they are.

Every day, every experience, every choice is an opportunity for awakening.

Making the leap from an unawakened life to an awakened one is possible with five core practices:

Coming back to the present moment
Connecting with something greater
Growing your trust
Embodying love
Holding openness

Like awakening itself, these practices are discussed and reflected upon by many thinkers and teachers, but they came to me through my personal lived experience.

Life took on a whole new meaning for me after my first awakening experience at eleven years old. I saw with new eyes the beauty all around me. Day after day I delighted in little things like the light of the afternoon sun falling on the trees, the magnificent colors of the lilies in the garden, and the vivid blue sky that expanded endlessly above. Life felt precious and magical. I appreciated just being alive.

This vibrant feeling of aliveness had first arrived after weeks of my desperate prayers to survive a rare childhood cancer I'd been diagnosed with. As my chemotherapy treatments continued, I made an interesting discovery: I could call back this feeling of aliveness if I concentrated on feeling my breath come in and out and letting my thoughts go. Somehow I just decided to stop my mind when it would go to any scary thoughts, worries, or what-ifs. When I stopped my mind and just breathed, I felt peace. I felt again that sense of, "Ah, here I am!" and I could take a deeper breath. During these times, a warm sensation filled my heart, and deep gratitude stirred in my being. After a while I started experiencing these moments without trying.

I continued to live in this present-moment awareness through my teenage years, after my treatments ended and my cancer was considered to be in remission. The spontaneous experiences of feeling fully alive became more and more frequent. In the morning after breakfast, I'd stand in front of the mirror and comb my hair. I knew what it felt like to have no hair, because I'd lost all of mine during chemotherapy treatments. Now my hair was thick and curly, and I was so grateful. After school, I'd come home, sit on the floor, and hold my cat, Chaz. Her warm body rubbed up against me, and her purring filled my being. Her eyes stared into mine. My body vibrated with love. My heart continued to feel full of thankfulness, and the feeling and knowing of "I am here" constantly swirled in and around me. *How lucky am I?* I frequently thought. (Interestingly, later, as an adult in my twenties, I had an anxiety attack because I actually didn't know how to think about the future. I realized future-thinking was okay and that I needed to learn to do it for basic life planning.)

My childhood experience showed me the power of the first awakening practice: coming back to the present moment. I also started to understand the power of our mind and the idea that we create our reality with it.

This acute sense of the present moment wasn't my only source of comfort during my treatments. I continued to feel overwhelming peace and a tangible presence, which I started to call "God," watching over me. I told no one about them, just as I had told no one about my prayers to live to be twenty. I just held on to them. I leaned into this feeling of deep peace, the knowing that I was going to be okay, and the oneness I felt with everything around me. I carried them with me through the five years of CT scans and follow-up tests and beyond.

Meister Eckhart, a fourteenth-century Christian mystic said, "[W]e must learn to maintain an inner solitude regardless of where we are and who we are with." I learned this truth as a child. But in my solitude, I discovered I actually wasn't alone. Facing my death, I awakened to my soul and a visceral sense of connection to some-thing greater than myself. Today the practice of connecting with something greater—and living from this connection—continues to support my ongoing awakening and give me great comfort.

In my early thirties, I was a senior account executive for Time Warner, a career I enjoyed. As a top advertising salesperson, I had won the sales-incentive trip and was headed to Costa Rica. These trips were always fun. Costa Rica was beautiful, and our accommodations were lush.

One of our day trips was whitewater rafting, and I felt uneasy before it even started. As I looked at the fast-moving waters, I felt even more trepidation.

We were moving through rapids categorized as level three in whitewater rafting terms. But the river was high due to recent rains, and the rapids were actually more like level four. The head of our raft was a member of Costa Rica's Olympic whitewater rafting team, and he was fearless. All the other boats in our group were going around the more treacherous rapids, but not ours. He led our eight-person boat right down the middle of each rapid. My hands were slipping as I tried to hold on to the handle in the back corner of the raft. My heart was racing. We hit a huge rapid, and I was suddenly thrown upward and then plunged into the water. Despite my life vest and helmet, I was pulled deep underwater.

I curled in a fetal position. Everything was dark, silent. I was completely alone. Terror coursed through my body.

This is it, I thought. *I am finally going to die.*

I felt the same as I had at eleven years old, going through chemotherapy and being so sick. I saw myself again as a tiny, skinny, frail girl with no hair lying in a hospital bed, alone and scared.

Then a bright, radiant white light surrounded my entire body. I heard a voice say loudly and clearly, "Living or dying is fine."

Just as it had when I was eleven, peace poured through my body, permeating every ounce of my being. I let go and surrendered to it. A deep trust, a knowing, came through me: I was going to be okay, no matter what happened next. Again, I felt a deep reassurance that I was not alone. Only this time, deep underwater, I didn't know whether being okay meant I was going to live or die. My body started to uncurl.

Next thing I remember, I was grabbed by my life vest and pulled onto a boat. I was in shock, frozen. I couldn't speak. I kept hearing we had to keep going down the river to get out.

Motionless, I got back into my spot on the raft and held on tightly. I prayed continuously going down the final rapids. *Please be with me, God. May I stay on this raft. Be with me.*

When we landed on shore, I repeatedly said, "Thank you, God." My body started to calm. I did not talk to anyone about what I had experienced in the waters of the river. I was exhausted.

What I learned that day in the deep swells of the Costa Rican river was another lesson—this time in trust. I was asked to accept what was happening instead of fighting it and to trust that I would be okay no matter what happened.

A few days later, in a taxi headed to our home in Minneapolis, I called my mother to tell her I was back. As I started to tell her about my rafting trip, she gasped and said, "Catherine, I dreamed I slipped into a river and almost drowned. And then I woke up."

My mother had never shared a dream with me before. And the day she'd had this dream was the very day I'd nearly drowned in Costa Rica. A chill went down my body.

Was her dream a coincidence? Or was it synchronicity that my mother, whom I consider my best friend, had known and felt what I had been through? I believe it was the latter. As a child, when I was able to live in the present moment, I'd felt a oneness with something greater. My mother's dream deepened my understanding of what that oneness meant: not only was I a part of something greater, but we are all connected to one another through it.

This near-death experience was a turning point in my adult life. Afterward I felt again a heightened sense of being alive, similar to what I'd felt as a young child when I practiced living in the present moment. Having faced death again, I was given a new lens through which to view life. I awakened into a deeper understanding of what it meant to be fully alive. As a result, I felt called to listen more deeply for guidance and to trust what it said.

I also knew with certainty I was done with my high-paying, glamorous corporate job, and I quit. I realized there were many paths beyond the corporate world. Having just had a dramatic lesson in trust, I longed for space and silence so I could hear my soul and my inner wisdom and discover which path I was being called to follow next. I carved out time daily to pray, meditate, and journal. Even though I did not know what my next steps would be, I trusted I was being guided, and I'd live into them. Even as family members questioned what I was doing, I kept listening deeply. Meanwhile, I picked up some part-time work and stayed open to any sign, promptings, and inner guidance that would tell me what the next steps on my path were.

Within a few months, my girlfriend Connie suggested I study theology and spiritual direction at St. Catherine University. I had never thought of graduate school, let alone studying theology. And yet this suggestion was perfect for me, given that I'd been obsessed with reading books on life, meaning, and purpose since my teenage years. I requested some materials about the school's theology program, and when they arrived, my body started physically shaking.

I prayed, "Is this the right step?"

I heard and felt a yes.

I didn't look back. I trusted the guidance and moved forward. My second awakening experience gave me a deeper understanding of trust. I discovered that my trust grew when I was able to accept whatever was happening, good or bad, without trying to control or change it, and when I created space to listen deeply for guidance.

My cell phone rang during dinner with friends. My husband had collapsed and was being taken to the hospital.

Panic rose in my chest, and I made my way to the emergency room, where doctors struggled to make sense of Scott's symptoms. Was he suffering a heart attack? An aortic dissection? A strange cardiac rhythm? While he was wheeled from room to room for different tests, I sat by myself in his ER room, gasping for air. The doctors ruled out an aortic dissection but still didn't know what was going on.

He was moved to the cardiac floor for observation. Soon after arriving there, Scott flatlined. Owen, my twenty-two-year-old son, ran down the hospital corridor to find a nurse. After what seemed like minutes, several nurses ran in, and seconds later the monitors showed a heartbeat again. Scott was then moved into the intensive care unit (ICU).

Breathe, I told myself on the second day Scott was in the ICU. I wanted to run from the terror rising in my body, from the fear bubbling up, but I knew I'd only drop into deeper suffering if I did. I decided in the moment not to let my mind run me. Instead, I chose to slow down my thoughts by focusing on the feel of my breath moving in and out of my body. I wanted the present moment to be my anchor.

For the next ten days, the outside world stopped, and my family's whole existence was within the walls of the ICU. Standing with me in the sterile hallways, the doctors said multiple times, "He is here. Most men die of this. We will figure this out." I tried to hold on to their reassurance and feel gratitude amid the fear within and around me. At times my mind took over, fear creeped in, panic rushed up and down my spine, and tears welled up in my eyes.

What gave me solace during that time was my practice of staying in the present moment. I'd focus on my breathing, feeling my lower abdomen expand on the in-breath and recede on the out-breath. As I walked down the hospital corridors, I focused on my body, the strength in my legs. As the days went by, the pull to live one moment at a time deepened. I focused on each day, moment to moment, and tried not to let my mind wander to the many possible what-ifs. And by choosing to live one moment at a time, I felt calmness in my heart and a grounding and comfort in my soul. I also felt again that deep sense of oneness and interconnectedness—with others and with something greater.

We eventually learned that Scott's heart had been damaged by cardiac sarcoidosis, a very rare heart condition that causes inflammation in the heart muscle and electrical damage to the whole heart.

Faced with the possible death of someone close to me, I saw that all that really matters in life is love. Everything else lost significance. The healing and grounding found in deep love felt and shared is what's most important. I'd already learned this lesson from the many hospice patients I companioned on their deathbeds. The only thing all these patients wanted was love—to feel love within and for those closest to them. Scott's brush with death reinforced this lesson for me.

After he was discharged, I found myself wanting to hold on to all the love I felt. I started exploring ways I could not just recover that feeling of love but also intentionally strengthen and expand it.

Today, seven years later, my husband is navigating a drug regimen of immunosuppressant pills and leading a pretty normal life. Choosing to live one day at a time, one moment at a time, is still a soothing balm for me. I've also continued my daily practice of cultivating embodied love. Even before I get out of bed in the morning, for example, I spend a few minutes feeling gratitude for life. I work on loving myself and sharing love with others. I also practice forgiveness, feeling into my heart center, and letting go of judgment.

As we navigate Scott's doctor appointments and the reality of his rare heart condition, I've also felt the power of holding openness. I've learned that when I stay open to whatever is happening in the moment and resist the urge to close down during difficult times, I'm able to keep my emotional balance and move with the flow of life instead of just reacting or going to emotional extremes. At the same time, I'm able to feel my feelings and the preciousness of life more deeply. Holding openness through life's challenges, no matter how difficult they may be, has only helped me feel more fully alive.

Periodically in my daily meditation practice, while I'm sitting in silence and stillness, I may feel a rumbling deep within. A pang of unease might come up. As I breathe into this unease, it becomes more present. I know I have the choice to feel and release it or to shut it down. Since I'm committed to holding openness, I choose the former. The practice of coming into the present moment helps me do that.

As I continue living through the coronavirus pandemic—and all the unrest, division, suffering, and death visible in the news and in our lives—intentionally holding openness continues to help me stay balanced and move with the flow of life, which in turn enables me to find ease and peace. I make the conscious choice to stay open to the mystery of life.

These five practices—coming back to the present moment, connecting with something greater, growing my trust, embodying love, and holding openness—have shaped and molded who I am and my understanding of being alive. I consciously practice and live into them daily.

They are also the core practices I keep coming back to as I work with clients. After years as a hospital and hospice chaplain, I felt an inner pull to help people feel more fully alive *right now* instead of waiting until the moment of their deaths. I started a private practice as an integrative spiritual consultant, providing one-on-one emotional, intuitive, and spiritual support for a variety of people. No matter what their circumstances, nearly all my clients begin finding more life and meaning as they begin using these five awakening practices.

Being human, we all get pulled into autopilot mode, engaging with others and the world solely from our ego mind. With these five practices, we can find our grounding again, remember who we are, and live more fully from our heart and soul each day as we navigate this terrain called life.

Each practice alone will allow you to feel more peace, ease, and spaciousness. But the practices also augment and build on each other. We start with simply coming back into just this moment, and from there we can open into deeper layers of awakening. Coming back into the present moment takes us out of our thinking mind and creates room for connecting with our soul and with something greater. That connection helps us grow our trust through accepting what is and through listening deeply. When we are present in the moment and not lost in our minds, we are able to feel love more acutely in our body, our heart, and our whole being. The relief of coming back to the present moment, along with a felt connection with something greater, a felt sense of trust, and a felt sense of love, enable us to hold openness through life's inevitable challenges. By staying open to all of life, we are able to live fully and love deeply.

In each of the following chapters, I'll give you different exercises, tools, and teachings that will help you live into each of these five practices every day. Each of the practices can be accessible to everyone, but not everyone will access it the same way. I've provided many different options so that you can find *your* way into each core practice—the way that fits your unique needs and capabilities. If one particular exercise doesn't work for you, try another, or you might try modifying the exercise a little bit to see if it works better for you that way. If you find one of the practices or exercises exacerbates a particular mental or physical health condition, don't do it. And please keep in mind that these practices are a complement to, not a replacement for, physical, mental, emotional, and spiritual health care from qualified professionals.

We don't have to wait until we're faced with our imminent death or with a dramatic life event to awaken. Everyday life gives us a lot of opportunities to awaken little by little. All of us have to navigate ups and downs, sorrows, and challenges. The question is, do we do so in a way that makes us feel shut down, tuned out, and closed off from ourselves and from life? Or do we want to do the opposite—open ourselves to being more fully present and alive?

You can choose to be present for your life and feel fully alive right now. Learning to do so is what everyday awakening is all about.

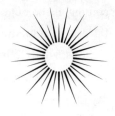

2

THE FIRST PRACTICE

Come Back to the Present Moment

RIGHT WHERE YOU ARE, right now, take a deep breath. Close your eyes for a minute, and feel your breath coming in and out of your body. Just breathe.

Can you notice the coolness of the air coming through your nostrils as you breathe in and the warmth of the air as you breathe out? Can you notice that when you breathe in the air turns and starts to go down into your chest? Notice how your chest and lower abdomen expand on the in-breath and recede on the out-breath.

When you breathe out, there are a few moments of space, stillness, before you take your next breath. Can you feel this?

Watch the ebb and flow of your breath for another minute or so. When you're ready, open your eyes.

You just experienced being in the present moment.

How did it feel?

Watching your breath coming in and out of your body is one way of coming back into the present moment. You could also watch your thoughts, feelings, actions, what your five senses are taking in, something in your environment, or your body's energy. What you choose to watch doesn't matter. What matters is that you are fully engaged in watching it. When you do that, you're fully in the present moment. And when you're in the present moment, you're not in your thinking mind.

The state of being fully in the present moment, fully in the here and now, can be called *presence*. Presence is found in the spaces between our thoughts.

When we make coming back to the present moment a regular practice, we can grow our ability to stay there for longer. Eventually, the feeling of the present moment can become our anchor. We naturally will move back into our thinking mind to live life— to go to appointments, dinners, meetings—but we no longer get lost in our thinking mind. When we are able to make the present moment our anchor, we're able to live in it more and more and awaken.

> [O]nly the present moment can make us free.
> That realization is the awakening.
> —Eckhart Tolle, A New Earth

Awakening into the Present Moment

Now, forty years later, as an adult, living a healthy life, the practice of coming back to the present moment is still as vital to me as it was when I was a child. I find ease, love, joy, and peace living from the present moment, and I'm attuned to noticing if I stray away. If

I can catch my mind wandering to the future or past—to a fear, a worry, a what-if—I breathe my way back in.

Many people are taken aback when they first experience how much their energy, feelings, and outlook can shift with this seemingly simple practice. Joe was one such person.

In our first visit, he talked about his highly successful corporate job, his travels, and his lucrative income. He worked nonstop and only occasionally enjoyed a beer with colleagues. He had been married for a few years and then divorced. His focus was on his career, money, and recognition. But something was missing. Joe had contacted me for an integrative counseling session because he felt a gnawing sense of loneliness and emptiness. He said he was feeling depressed and numb.

"I don't know if I can keep living like this," he said. "I feel little to nothing. All I do is work. Is this really what life is all about?"

The more we talked, the more I sensed that Joe had been living almost exclusively in his mind.

"You also have a heart and a soul, and they're yearning to open," I told him.

Then I led Joe in a five-minute breathing exercise. Afterward his eyes welled up with tears. "I am here," he said. "I haven't felt peace like this in so long." He buried his head in his hands and cried.

On his next visit, Joe declared, "I've been practicing breathing and meditating, and my whole understanding of life has changed. I'm experiencing some moments of peace for the first time in my life. I'm happier. Even my family is noticing that I have changed."

If you are craving more of a sense of aliveness, a richness, a deepening experience of love and joy, it is possible. It is possible to have moments of presence in which your mind stops, and peace enters. Trust me: you can start training yourself to notice and cultivate them just by coming back to the present moment, right here, right now.

Breathe in Peace, Breathe out Stress

Here is the breath exercise I led Joe in. Try it and see what you feel.

Sit or lie in a comfortable position.

Let your shoulders drop. Feel your breath coming in and out of your body. If you are feeling any tightness or tension, just breathe into that area for a moment.

Now focus on your breath—your in-breath, your out-breath—letting your body soften and relax for the next minute.

On your next in-breath, imagine breathing in peace through the top of your head. See and feel it flowing down through your head, neck, shoulders, chest, abdomen, hips, legs, knees, and feet.

On your out-breath, breathe out any stress through your feet. Or you can visualize stress like gray smoke leaving your body.

Keep breathing in peace, imagining it flowing through your entire body from the top down, and then breathing out any stress. If your mind wanders, just come back to your breath. Continue breathing in peace and breathing out any stress for five minutes.

Building the Presence Habit

Practicing coming back to the present moment may at first not seem like a big deal. But over time it can have a profound effect, especially if you keep doing it and thus build your ability to stay in the present moment for longer and longer.

The number-one problem I hear from people new to this practice is that they just can't seem to find time in their daily lives to do it. They love the exercises during our session, but then they say they have a hard time picking up the practice again on their own.

When I hear this, I suggest they not think of coming into the present moment as a formal practice; instead, they should think of it as a good habit. Forming a new habit typically takes only about sixty-six days. To get into the habit of coming into the present moment, I suggest they find one simple exercise they enjoy and can commit to doing for just five minutes each day for one week. After one week, they can check in with themselves and see how they feel. If they're not feeling more spaciousness, stillness, and peace, or if they're not enjoying their chosen exercise, they can try another one.

Some people successfully start their new presence habit by linking the practice to an everyday activity. For example, in the morning while you're drinking your cup of tea or coffee, turn off all external distractions, like your phone and other electronic devices. Give your full attention to what you're feeling, smelling, and sensing. Hold your cup. Feel its warmth. Smell the aroma of your coffee or tea. Take a sip and fully enjoy the taste in just this moment.

Maybe you have a window in your kitchen or room. If so, look out the window, just noticing what is there. Be fully present while you drink your coffee and look out the window for a couple of minutes.

You can practice presence while eating your lunch. Hold your sandwich or your salad bowl. Notice all the colors, smells, and textures as you are fully present in the moment with your food. Take a bite and savor it. Spend at least a few minutes being fully present as you eat.

Even walking to the bathroom can be an opportunity to practice. As you get up from your chair, feel the weight of your body in your legs. Feel the floor supporting your body. Notice your breath coming in and out of your lungs as you walk.

Any everyday moment can become a moment of presence. And as you continue to practice, you likely will start experiencing spontaneous moments of presence. Maybe you notice a surge of energy moving in your body, a warmth fills your chest, or a strong emotion of gratitude or love fills your being. Maybe you feel the softness of the wind touch your cheek. Your mind might slow down and maybe even stop. Perhaps a sense that there is something more, beyond this physical body, emerges.

These moments of presence might seem short and fleeting, but they're valuable. And they don't have to be rare. All you need to do is keep practicing.

Using the Senses to Come Back to the Present Moment

Coming into the present moment doesn't require a special time, setting, or effort. You can easily practice it throughout your day, during seemingly mundane moments, just by tuning in to your five senses.

First, spend a minute or two just focusing on your breath—breathing in and breathing out.

When you are ready, spend a minute noticing what you *see*.

Next, spend a minute noticing what you *hear*.

Take one minute to notice what you *feel*. Be in your body and breathe in and breathe out. Let everything else drop away.

Notice for the next minute what you *smell*.

Then notice for the next minute what you *taste*.

Finally, come back to your breath. Just focus on breathing in and breathing out for a few moments.

How are you feeling as you finish this short practice? Take a few minutes and write down what you noticed. Any new insights?

Minding the Mind

I regularly hear clients say, "My mind is running me. I'm exhausted. I want to slow down." Others say to me, "So this is life? I've mastered my job. I'm at the top, but I feel empty, depleted. I'm craving room to breathe."

The reason many people feel like they're living on autopilot is that their reality is grounded in their mind. They live in their mind, plugging along, not conscious of the preciousness of this moment, of breathing, and of being alive.

Maybe you notice that you can't stop your endless thoughts and mind chatter. Maybe you start the day with thoughts on what it will include, such as appointments, errands, and visits, and you feel overwhelmed before you even get started. Your thoughts have energy, and when your mind is running your life, you're often living in a stress response, with cortisol, a stress hormone, coursing through your body.

Our world acknowledges individuals who are brilliant, innovative, and highly intellectual. Most of us are conditioned to focus on and develop our minds, increase our intelligence, and see life through a mental framework. This mental framework is often devoid of an emotional, energetic, or spiritual lens. Living only in our minds keeps us from fully experiencing what it means to be alive, and open to the wonder of life. Our minds might bring us success, achievement, and value in the world, but if we don't feel the beauty of being alive, the vibration of life, the energy, love, and joy pulsing through us and around us, something is missing.

When we live in our thinking ego mind, we are at its mercy. Our mind is attached to form, identity, desires, and passions, and these attachments run who we are. We ruminate over the past or the future. We often embody judgment, separation, a feeling of less than, and we shut down, avoid, try to control, and try to not feel. When our mind is running the show, we cannot experience a felt sense of spaciousness, stillness, or aliveness. We lose ourselves.

Some people tell me they are so used to living in their mind that they can't stop their endless thoughts and mind chatter for even just a few minutes in order to come into the present moment. When this happens, I suggest that maybe instead of fighting against their thoughts, they should try watching those thoughts.

At the beginning of this chapter, you took a few moments to watch your breath. You can also do the same thing with your thoughts: you can step back and witness where your mind goes. When you do, you're experiencing *awareness*, the state of having stepped back from your thinking mind in order to witness your thoughts and feelings. When you choose to watch what your mind is doing, you shift out of autopilot and come back to the present moment. Your mind slows down, and its grip on you loosens. You can feel the fullness of being alive. You can feel the beauty, joy, and peace that is within and around you. You can drop into silence and timelessness and open into deeper layers of consciousness. From there, you can start to run your life instead of letting your mind run you.

We live in a fast-paced world that is crowded with news, opinions, chaos, and upheaval. We are making a choice each day about how we live. And if we are not choosing to move out of our busy, chattering mind, we are subconsciously choosing a path of unawareness.

Freedom arises when you understand that you are the master of your mind.

The ultimate question is, are you the master of your mind, or is your mind the master?

Witnessing Thoughts

Sit in a comfortable position. Focus on your breath, breathing in and breathing out.

Notice what is arising in your mind and body. Whatever is arising in this moment, just be with it.

Can you watch your mind, being the witnessing presence? Can you watch the thoughts come and then watch them go, as if they were just clouds drifting across the sky?

If your mind goes to a thought of the past or future, consciously come back to your breath. Focus just on breathing in and breathing out.

Let your body soften and relax, breathing in and breathing out.

You can spend as much time as you wish witnessing your thoughts and feelings as they arise and dissipate. If you are new to this, start with five minutes. When you're ready to stop, bring your focus back to your breath, breathing in and breathing out.

Out of the Mind and into the Body

The deep peace I first encountered as an eleven-year-old didn't come from the tangible, material world. Nor did it come from my mind. It came through my body. Unlike our minds, our bodies are always in the present moment. So, when we find ourselves too caught up in our thinking ego minds, an easy way back to the present moment is to tune in to our breath and its movement in our body.

This meditation usually takes about ten minutes, but take whatever time is right for you. Definitely feel free to slow down and linger at different points if it feels right.

Sit or lie in a comfortable position. You may want to close your eyes so you are not distracted.

Bring your attention to your breath, breathing in and breathing out.

Now tune in to your body. Be open and curious. Open to just what is, with no judgment.

Next, you are going to bring attention to each part of your body.

First notice if you have any tension or tightness anywhere in your body. If you do, just breathe into that tense area for a moment.

Now take a minute and tune in to what you are thinking and feeling. Are you calm, restless, grounded, agitated? Notice what is going on without judging or trying to change anything.

Now bring your attention back to your breath, breathing in and breathing out.

Become aware of where you feel your breath most. It might be in your nose, chest, stomach, or elsewhere. Breathe in deeply and notice the breath as it fills your body. Witness your body expanding on the in-breath and receding on the out-breath.

Bring your attention to the top of your head, then, in turn, to your face, forehead, eyes, cheeks, jaw, and mouth. Whatever you are experiencing in this moment, allow it to just be.

Now move your attention down into your neck and shoulders, noticing if you have any tightness there.

Move your attention now into your arms, elbows, wrists, hands, fingers. Notice any sensations you feel. Just feel what's there.

Now move your attention down into your chest, your heart area, your beating heart. Continue feeling your body as it breathes for you.

Invite your heart to soften and expand. Feel warmth and softening in your heart area. Spend a few moments paying attention to this warmth, feeling it and feeling love within your body.

Now move your attention into your stomach. Notice what you feel in this area. Do you feel a sense of calmness, tightness, or something else? This is the area of your body where you digest life. What are you feeling here? Open to what is present here in this moment.

Now move your attention to your hips, your legs, your thighs, your knees, your ankles, and your feet. Feel how each part of your body is connected to the next.

Feel the vibration of aliveness coursing through your body.

And now let your attention rest again on your breath, breathing in and breathing out. Feel your body expand on the in-breath and recede on the out-breath.

And now bring your awareness back to the present moment. Let your breathing deepen. Feel your body being supported as you breathe in and out.

When you are ready, you can gently open your eyes.

Negative Thoughts Don't Have to Run Us

When your mind is in the driver's seat, it can sometimes take you for a wild ride. It is easy to think negatively, and negative thoughts can easily take over and dominate your life. Negative thoughts turn on your body's stress response.

Perhaps a friend or family member says a negative comment to you or cuts you off midsentence. Your mind immediately grabs on to the negative words, and a feeling like irritation, anger, or anxiety arises, prompting you to start replaying the experience in your mind. Then more feelings start bubbling up. Your thoughts are the energy that triggers the feelings, and pretty soon you're swinging back and forth from thoughts to feelings. You've turned on the stress response in your body by thought alone, and your mind will keep it going.

Sound familiar? This response is known as a limbic loop, and it happens to all of us.

> *Your brain is like Velcro for negative experiences*
> *and Teflon for positive ones.*
> —Rick Hanson, PhD, and Richard Mendius, MD, Buddha's Brain

Our minds are naturally wired to focus on the negative. The term for this is *negativity bias*. Since prehistoric times, humans have survived by learning to anticipate worst-case scenarios. Our brains have evolved over thousands of years to look for the negative in order to survive.

When you're stuck in a limbic loop, you are strengthening the neural pathways, or series of connected neurons, in your brain that watch for negative experiences. These pathways send signals between the various parts of the brain that are together known as the limbic system. The longer the limbic loop continues, the stronger those neural pathways become, which only further reinforces the loop. And the stronger the limbic loop becomes, the more hold our negative thoughts will have on us.

Coming back to the present moment and choosing to become a witness to our thoughts and feelings will disrupt our limbic loops.

Imagine you're feeling fearful. Instead of letting your mind run with that fear, you could take a step back from it. From that place of awareness, you can say out loud or silently to yourself, "Oh, there I go again. I am ruminating about a fearful thought." Naming the negative thought and identifying the feeling will start to calm your nervous system.

From there, you can refocus on the present moment by taking a deep breath and bringing your attention to your breathing or a part of your body, such as the energy moving in your hands. When you do that, you can't think at the same time. Your mind slows, and a feeling of spaciousness can enter.

At this point you can feel the fear that is present. Keep breathing as you feel it. It takes courage to breathe into whatever feeling is arising. But as you feel your feelings and breathe into them, they will start to dissipate.

The final step is saying a positive affirmation or bringing to mind a positive image or memory. By marinating in the good—in positive thoughts—you create healthy new neural pathways in your brain. Building and reinforcing new neural pathways will keep old limbic loops from reactivating and keep new limbic loops from forming.

We have the power to not let our negative thoughts, our negative ruminations, run our lives. We can choose what we think and feel, thereby shaping our lives daily.

A conscious being holds on nowhere.
—*Ram Dass,* Polishing the Mirror

Retrain Your Negative-Thinking Mind

Here is a step-by-step version of the process described above. The next time negative thoughts trigger a stress response, you can use these steps to interrupt the limbic loop.

1. Become aware. Ask yourself, "What am I thinking?"
2. Identify your negative thought.
3. Come back to your body. Your body is always in the present moment.
4. Take a few minutes to breathe. Just feel your breath coming in and out of your body. Or you may want to feel the energy pulsing in your hands. When you focus on your breath or the energy pulsing in your hands, your thinking mind stops.
5. Now name the feeling you are feeling.
6. Where in your body do you feel that feeling? Locate that feeling in your body. Maybe you feel it in your head, your chest, or your stomach area. Maybe you feel it elsewhere.
7. Breathe into the part of your body holding the feeling. Let yourself feel what is there for at least a few minutes. Feelings are not permanent, and by feeling them they will start to move and dissipate.
8. Shift your attention to your lower belly. Put your hand on it and breathe deeply.
9. Come back to the negative thought you identified in step 2. Replace it with a positive thought—for example, "I am strong and taking one day at a time."
10. Go to a positive memory. Feel the good feelings that arise with that memory. Take those feelings into your body and savor them.

11. Return to the present moment by focusing again on your breathing. Stay here, in the present moment, with your breath, and enjoy the peace, joy, and other sensations that arise.

Turn Suffering into Awakening

When we're suffering, our tendency to constantly move in and out of our thinking ego mind becomes more noticeable. Clinging to our mind and its many thoughts about what has happened in the past or might happen in the future only adds many layers of additional suffering.

In Buddhist teachings, suffering is compared to a pair of arrows. The first arrow is what actually happens; it is the things that are out of our control and cause our suffering. The second arrow is how we handle those things—how we usually ruminate, worry, and become engulfed by fear. The second arrow accentuates the suffering caused by the first arrow. Fortunately, this second arrow is something we can control and regulate.

We can choose to cultivate presence while navigating suffering. We can choose to come into the present moment and be present with our suffering instead of shutting down.

It might seem like choosing to be in just this moment, amid our pain and unrest, would exacerbate our suffering. But I have found the opposite is true: Coming back to the present moment provides great relief. A sense of the preciousness of life can surface when we enter into our suffering rather than trying to avoid it. It often takes suffering to open us to a sense of presence that is always here for us. And it is through the hardships that we can start to learn to live deeply in this moment.

Two roads diverged in a wood, and I—
I took the one less traveled by,
And that has made all the difference.
—Robert Frost, "The Road Not Taken"

When we're suffering, our feelings can be a doorway into the present moment. It takes courage, strength, and resilience to be present with and feel into our feelings at such times. It would be easier to distract ourselves with our phones, TV, and the news, or stuff our feelings down. But when we continually push down or deny our feelings, they get buried deep within us, only to be triggered at another time. Or they get stuck in our bodies and, over time, transform into illness and disease. I have been there and denied feelings while navigating suffering. It may temporarily feel good, but feeling them later makes them feel even worse.

When we do feel our feelings, they shift and move and drop, and freedom and space have room to enter. There is now room to take a deeper breath. Silence arises and stillness surfaces, and a deeper felt sense of presence emerges within us.

In this felt spaciousness in the present moment, you might feel as though you're stepping out of time. In this felt sense of time-lessness, there is more space to breathe and experience what is present, including the tenderness of the moment. You may notice and feel the beauty of a sunset or of kids laughing and giggling. A smile may come into your eyes as you touch into and feel the preciousness of life. Often a knowing arises that "*Ah*, I am here!"

Feeling our feelings brings us back into the present moment, and there we can face, enter, and release our feelings and suffering. And when we do that, our suffering becomes our awakening.

Self-Soothing Practice

Here is an exercise to come back into the present moment when you are suffering or feeling unrest.

I invite you to close your eyes.

Place your hands over your heart area and breathe.

Let your body soften and relax. Feel your breath, breathing in and breathing out.

Feel the warmth of your hands over your heart area.

Feel your heart soften.

Breathing in and out.

Notice what you are feeling.

Name the feeling.

Notice where you feel it in your body.

Continue breathing in and breathing out.

Now say a loving-kindness phrase, such as, "May I be at peace," or, "Be with me."

Breathe in and breathe out.

Spend a few minutes or longer just breathing in and out.

And when you are ready, you can gently open your eyes.

Feeling Fully Alive While Dying

When I became a hospice chaplain, I saw many patients realize the same thing I had as a child: coming into the present moment can help us face even the gravest life-and-death situations. Again and again, I saw dying patients choose to stay in the present moment instead of getting lost in their thinking minds and the fear their thoughts could generate. They opened to what was happening and felt deeply instead of turning away from their pain and difficult feelings. As a result, they experienced love, joy, and a feeling of full aliveness even as their lives were ending.

As a Buddhist dedicated to mindfulness, my patient Bill had been practicing coming into the present moment throughout his life. When he was dying from ALS (amyotrophic lateral sclerosis), he wanted to continue learning what living in the present moment really meant. Sometimes during my visits he'd hold my hand, and we'd just sit together in silence, breathing and taking in the preciousness of the moment.

One day I arrived to find him sitting up in his bed. He gave me a faint smile. He had lost the ability to speak and communicated to people by looking into a computer screen that then spoke his words.

"I am alive," he said via the automated voice. Tears rolled down his face. "I want to keep opening and growing to the very last moment. I want to teach my children how to die well."

An electrifying calmness filled the room. His sense of aliveness was palpable. His body was deteriorating and not long for this world, and yet his spirit was bright. My heart expanded and opened and my own tangible sense of presence sharpened as I sat with him.

Because he was able to live in the present moment, Bill only became more vibrantly alive every day despite his physical decline. In his final days, being fully present allowed him to move beyond his mind and live free of fear. In doing so, he was able to feel the deep love of his wife and children, who were by his bedside.

Like Bill, my mother-in-law, Karen, also showed me how living in the present moment can help us even as we face the end of our life. She had been battling pancreatic cancer for one year, and the doctors had said there was nothing more they could do for her. She entered hospice care in her home.

One hot, sunny Friday afternoon, she invited my husband and me to join her in her bedroom. At that time she was still walking around, highly functional, and eating. We all sat down together on her bed.

She smiled, looked deeply in our eyes, and said, "I am going to teach you about death and dying. I am ready. I am not afraid."

My eyes widened. I sensed no fear or unrest on her part. Instead, I felt her acute sense of the present moment. Her presence was like a luminous light shining through her. I'd been practicing living in the present moment for most of my life, but here with Karen, I understood on an even deeper level what living fully felt and looked like.

Three days later she was actively dying. In her final hours, her breath became shallow, yet I felt peace throughout the room. Her deep sense of presence only magnified her aliveness as she was about to leave this earth.

Both Bill and Karen could have suffered greatly as they faced the end of their lives. Instead, they chose to stay in the present moment, and as they did, their potential suffering became their awakening. Their choice to live in the present moment allowed them to feel fully alive even while dying. This is the power and practice of coming into the present moment.

Practicing Presence

This exercise is a short yet powerful way to come into the present moment and practice presence.

Bring your attention to your breath, breathing in and breathing out. Then say out loud, "I am presence."

Put your hands over your heart area. Feel the warmth of your hands fill your being and allow ease to fill your heart.

Fully Present and Fully Alive in This Moment

As I was sitting in my home office, looking out the glass-framed window, a large white egret swooped by and headed toward the nearby lake. A deep feeling of being just in this moment came through me. My heart skipped a beat as I marveled at the sight of this bird several feet from my window.

Minutes later several squirrels ran across the roof and leaped onto a tree branch that looked like it could barely hold them. Then they scurried to the trunk of the tree and ran down it. And a few minutes later, a red cardinal landed on another branch of the same tree, making eye contact with me, staring me down for a solid minute.

A sense of wonderment ran through my veins, snapping me out of my thinking mind. I'd been lost in deep thought about the coronavirus pandemic and what had been happening in the Twin Cities during the Derek Chauvin trial. The sense of unease and uncertainty, which had been floating in the cool morning air and drifting toward me through the open window, dropped away. I felt the aliveness of being fully present in the moment. And in that moment, I was able to witness the many creatures, so full of life, parading within feet of my window.

My identification with my thinking mind lifted for a moment. A stillness, a spaciousness, and peace surfaced. I felt connected to the egret, the squirrels, and the cardinal.

When we come into the present moment, we can drop into our soul. A door opens, our lens widens, and we can open into oneness with all of life.

Sitting in my office, I put my hand over my heart and felt love moving through my body. Then I grabbed my coffee and took a sip before my first Zoom call. I heard my daughter yell out the back door for our dog Bella, who was chasing squirrels and running laps around the yard. A flock of geese in a V-shaped formation flew over, squawking.

I smiled, feeling love and gratitude.

Coming into the present moment allows us to experience such moments of awe, wonder, and interconnectedness. Experiencing being present right now, feeling our heart beating, our breath coming in and out of our body, we open and feel more alive.

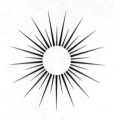

3

THE SECOND PRACTICE

Connect with Something Greater

HAVE YOU EVER HIT A wall and cried out for help? Have you realized you were at the end of your human efforts and needed help? It may feel like a burning sensation welling up within.

This is what I felt going through intensive treatments and multiple surgeries as a child. I was searching for help and longing for comfort. I started praying fervently to "God," the only name I had for something greater at the time.

After praying again and again, one late afternoon I suddenly felt a deep stillness and peace—a peace that seemed "not of this world," as Jesus said. It also felt like something greater was present with me. I felt a tangible sense of companionship. Feeling that presence of God helped carry me through the darkest time of my life.

When we move out of our fast-chattering thinking mind to just this moment, we drop from our minds into our heart; we open the door to stillness, space, deep peace—and maybe even something more. In the stillness between our thoughts, we can open into our soul.

When I speak of the soul, I'm referring to each person's unique essence. It is the energetic center of our physical being. Our soul is singular and unmatched in the world. It is timeless and eternal.

Touching our soul, we can experience a felt sense of oneness and interconnectedness with all. In this oneness, we may experience something greater, something beyond—an energy that is expansive and limitless and cannot be contained. We no longer feel separate and alone.

My first experience of something greater came suddenly, and I was under duress. Maybe you've touched into your soul and a felt sense of something greater when facing an upheaval. Yet you do not need to have a dramatic, life-changing event to open to something greater. You can choose to connect with your soul and with something greater right now.

Open into Your Soul

When Joe, whom you met in the previous chapter, started practicing coming back to the present moment, he found some moments of stillness. In that stillness, he suddenly realized he was a spirit, a soul, within a body.

It's easy for us to lose our connection with our soul, the home of our deep connection with something greater, when our thinking ego mind takes over our lives. We can't think our way into our soul. The way to find it is to come back to the present moment, to presence, and feel it in the spaciousness and stillness that's beyond the thinking ego mind. It takes mindfulness, strength, intention, and practice to stay in our soul and to see others as souls as well.

The difference between someone living from their mind and someone living from their soul is noticeable. When you're in the presence of a truly soul-filled person, you feel a light and love emanate from them. There is no sensation of their thinking ego mind. A few years ago, the Dalai Lama came to our town to give a talk. I was able to stand within a few feet of him for a moment. I marveled at his gentle, kind, loving energy. It felt like a breath of clean, pure, fresh air. It touched my heart and left me wanting to open and feel more. He was living from his soul, and I could feel it in my own soul and body.

> *The soul unfolds itself, like a lotus of countless petals.*
> —Kahlil Gibran, The Prophet

Every day we can choose where we are living from: our thinking ego mind or our soul. Can you live less out of your mind and more out of your soul? To do so, you need to notice when you are spending too much time in the mind and then choose to come back to the stillness of the present moment. There you can once again open into your soul.

Follow the Energy

This exercise will help you experience your energy—the life force pulsing through your body. Unaffected by your thoughts and feelings, this energy is your true essence and being—your soul. The more you take time to tune in and feel your energy, the easier it becomes, the more connected you'll feel to your soul, and the more alive you will feel. Tuning in to this life energy can also help you in those inevitable moments of confusion, doubt, unease, and anxiety.

First, let go of your thinking, worrying, procrastinating mind—the mind that plays multiple scenarios at one time. Remind yourself, "I am not my mind."

Next take a deep breath. Then another. Breathe deeply, becoming more and more aware of your breath coming in and out of your body. This will slow down your mind. It might take several deep breaths, but soon you'll begin to feel calm and present.

Now allow yourself to become still and quiet—still in the body, quiet in the mind.

In this space, feel your energy vibrating within your body.

Now say, "I am presence."

Notice what you feel.

Can feel your soul vibrating within you?

What do you feel in just this moment?

Continue breathing in and breathing out.

Feel the energy moving throughout your body. Let the sensation of energy within you reorient you. Let it help you feel fully alive again.

Spend the next few minutes feeling your life energy moving within as you breathe in and breathe out.

You Don't Have to Call It God

In my first few classes in graduate theology school, the professors asked, "What do you believe?" The emphasis was not on accepting a particular belief, understanding, or words but rather, "What do you believe in and why?"

I found this question so freeing. Having been raised Lutheran, I'd felt like I had to unquestionably embrace the creeds and confessions that were part of Sunday services. Now theology professors were giving me permission to explore all the facets of "faith." I was allowed to discover what beliefs and ideas resonated with me as I delved into the history of ancient civilizations and the roots of why and how religious and spiritual traditions came into form.

I see my soul, my essence, as grounded in oneness with something larger than myself. I most often call that "something greater" *God* or *the Divine.* Yet there's a whole range of other words that fit too—like *Source, Oneness, God, Allah, Great Spirit, the Infinite Field, love* or *Love, universal energy, a higher power, the quantum field.* The vast range of religious and spiritual traditions across the world all have different names for this something greater, and each name speaks to particular understanding of it. (If you find discord with this last thought, look up the term *religious pluralism,* another eye-opening concept I learned about in graduate theology school.) Each of these terms might be accurate, but each is also limited. It reflects just one perspective, one aspect, or one kind of experience of the greater something. The more I walk with people who are exploring their faith, meaning, and purpose and wanting to feel more fully alive, the more I think our words can only begin to touch on what that something greater is like. The whole of it is ultimately unnamable.

If you're just getting used to the idea of being part of something larger or greater than yourself, don't worry about what to call it. Don't get hung up on what others call it either. Language is limiting.

What's important is to be open to the feeling of it. Where, when, and how have you felt a sense of being connected to something greater, a sense of being interconnected with others, a sense that you're not alone even when you seem to be? If you can, recall a time you felt this way. Maybe you were on an evening walk, watching the sun set over the water. Or perhaps you were walking on a lakeside path, and you were greeted by a family of small birds scurrying toward the water. Or maybe you were outside and felt a warm breeze carrying a fragrant lilac smell and saw small flowers floating in the air.

As you picture that scene, can you open again to the feeling tone in your body, to a resonance with something more? What does it feel like? A sense of energy? A deep knowing? A glimmer of something beyond? A sense that there's a presence with you?

Again, don't worry about the language. Just feel it.

Maybe you experience a deep pulling of *ah*. Maybe you feel a sense of something bigger, and maybe an expanded, fuller breath comes in. Maybe you breathe in the preciousness of just this moment. Maybe you feel like you're settling into a deeper, fuller space within yourself.

Perhaps any held fear drops away, and you just know that in this moment all is okay. A wonderment comes through you, or a pulsing aliveness moves through your body. You feel an interconnectedness with all. A feeling of oneness and warmth fills your body.

Or maybe a feeling of coming home surfaces, the mirror is clear, and you understand why you are here.

I experience this feeling as an internal vibration that quivers within me. I also experience it as love. To me, our soul, our essence, feels like love; the felt sense of oneness and interconnectedness I feel through my soul feels like love; the something greater feels like love.

These are all examples of what something greater could feel like. What does it feel like to you?

Feel into Something Greater

The feelings or experience of something larger can arise spontaneously or under certain conditions, such as when you're spending time in nature. You can also create space for them. Here is a short breathing exercise to help you move into your body, heart, and soul and feel what is already present.

Relax your body, perhaps sitting in a chair or comfortably standing. Notice your breath coming in and out through your nostrils. Breathe in and breathe out.

Slowly let go of all external and internal distractions and just breathe. Let there be room for silence and stillness.

Breathing in, feel your belly expand on the in breath. And breathing out, feel your belly recede. Can you feel the cool air flow through your nostrils as you breathe in and the warm air as you breathe out? On your breath in, can you feel the air turn and go down into your chest?

As thoughts come into your mind, let them pass, like white clouds moving across the blue sky. Come back to your breath, breathing in and breathing out, one breath at a time.

In this moment, just notice what is.

Next, spend a minute noticing what you see.

Then notice what you hear.

And then notice what you feel.

Continue breathing in and breathing out.

Gently bring yourself back to your breath when your mind wanders.

Your fast-chattering mind will slow, and your soul will have room to expand and just be.

Spend as much time as you wish here, breathing in and breathing out and feeling your soul. Notice what else you may be feeling or experiencing.

What does it feel like? Just feel whatever is arising. Just be open. Just feel and experience what you are experiencing. If words arise, that is fine and then come back to what you are feeling.

You don't have to call it God. Let words drop away. Be open to the experience.

Let your body soften and relax as you breathe in and breathe out for the next few minutes.

Opening the Door to Something Greater— Just a Little

If you've read this far, you may be thinking, *I'm not sure I believe in anything more.*

My message to you is, be open.

When you are open to the idea of something greater, even just a little, you will experience a greater sense of aliveness, love, and joy. Might there just be more to this thing called life and being alive? Maybe there *is* more than what our analytical, intellectual brain can figure out. Spiritual traditions throughout the world share mystical stories and teachings. All dial in to the everyday mystic who connects with something more, something greater, and a sense of union and oneness. Maybe all these stories are speaking to a common experience that we all can experience too.

> [T]he true self is in the middle of our chest, in our spiritual heart.
> So, to get from ego to the true self I said: "I am loving awareness."
> —Ram Dass

One of my clients, Jane, told me how heartbroken she was when her thirteen-year-old dog, Molly, died. Because I believe all beings, including animals, have souls and are interconnected in a felt oneness, I suggested she be open to any dreams or signs from Molly. Jane wasn't sure there was something greater, but she was willing to be open.

In our next visit a week later, Jane said, "I've been excited to talk with you! I dreamed the other night that Molly was young and running in a green field. There was a half rainbow in the sky, and I knew she was okay. The next day my mother also had a dream of Molly. She dreamed that Molly was with her deceased dog, and they were together and happy.

"I marveled at the synchronicity of both of us having this dream. But I've still been praying to God and saying, 'I need a big sign to get the message.'

"Then you would not believe what happened. Yesterday, when we were leaving our cabin up north, Ben, my husband, and I decided to go for one last swim before we got in the car to head back to the city. We grabbed inner tubes and jumped off the dock. As we were enjoying the water and talking, we heard and saw a loon in the distance. Next thing you know, this loon popped up in the water between us. It was four feet away. I could have petted it. For about five minutes, it just stared at me. I felt scared, and then I just trusted. It was hauntingly beautiful and regal. Ben then started to swim to shore, and this loon swam next to him.

"I know this was a sign. I looked up the sacred meaning of loon, and it is about opening to dreams and their messages and the messages from beyond. I now know Molly is okay. I feel better. I don't feel alone anymore."

We sat in silence and smiled at each other. A knowing passed through us: we are in fact not alone. Jane's experiences convinced her there is something greater in the universe. And if we are open, it has messages for us.

When we connect with something greater, we don't feel alone. We open into a feeling of expansiveness and oneness. Feeling this interconnectedness with something greater and with all living beings, we open and become more fully alive.

Reach Out to Something Greater

Sit quietly and let your body relax.

Notice if you are holding any tension or tightness and just breathe into that area for a minute.

Put your hands over your heart area and just breathe.

Breathing in and breathing out, let your body soften and relax.

Now invite help in. You might say, "Help me. Be with me. Fill me with your love, light, and peace."

Just be open.

Receive.

Allow spaciousness and stillness to enter.

If your mind wanders, it is okay—just come back to your breath.

Breathe in and breathe out.

Let go.

Receive.

Spend the next five minutes being open and receiving.

Afterward, take a moment to reflect on your experience. What was it like for you? What did you notice? What did you feel? Maybe make a note of it in a journal. And be open to whatever comes and whatever you may experience next.

_____

Connecting with Something Greater through Prayer

After an emergency surgery, Jill had spent a couple of years dealing with debilitating pain and an array of body imbalances. I worked with her as she navigated the ups and downs with her health. Together we unearthed her family-of-origin story; worked to counter the effects of growing up in a stressful home that was full of negativity and fear; and reframe her negative, critical thoughts, which caused her to live on high alert.

Jill's deepest desire was to feel a oneness with the Divine—to drop out of her thinking ego mind and into her heart and soul, where the felt oneness and connection with all resides. One day she told me that she'd had an aha moment.

"While making some food in the kitchen, I pleaded to God, 'Please come down. Be with me. Let me open to your presence.'" As she'd continued walking around the kitchen, she suddenly felt a deep sensation of love fill her heart. This strong, palpable feeling of love and warmth spread throughout her body, which softened and relaxed.

A knowing surfaced in that moment of felt presence: Jill realized she was not alone.

Though the sense of warmth and love eventually subsided, Jill now knows that it exists. On challenging days, she can lean with more confidence into her knowing that there is something greater.

If you knew Who walks beside you on the way that
you have chosen, fear would be impossible.
—A Course in Miracles

Jill experienced a feeling and knowing of something greater by putting out her desires through prayer and invocation and then listening. You can intentionally call in a connection with something greater in the same way, even if you've never prayed before.

Prayer Practice to Open

You don't need to be religious or spiritual to pray. If you're new to prayer and would like to try calling in a conscious connection with something greater, you can do so with this two-part prayer practice.

Part 1: Call Out to Something Greater

Come back to the present moment and breathe.

As you come into your heart and soul, reach out and talk to something beyond you. In your mind or heart, either silently or out loud, say whatever comes into your heart.

If no words come, you can try any or all of these: *Thank you. Please forgive me. Be with me. Pour your healing spirit through me. Fill me with your love and light and peace. Help me open to your presence, your wisdom, your guidance. Lead me and guide me every step of my path. Protect me and my family. I pray for my family and friends. Be with me. Thank you.*

Part 2: Let Go and Listen

After you've called out and shared your heart, let go, be still, and listen.

Let there be space and ease within and around you. Choose to just be and allow. Don't make an effort. Just let your heart and mind soften.

Breathing into the present moment, let any thoughts float by. If your mind wanders, come back to your body and breath.

As you continue coming back to the present moment, a feeling of spaciousness and stillness will surface, giving you room to hear.

In this space and stillness, you may receive guidance, a knowing, a felt sense of something more, or more clarity on why you are here on this earth and breathing right now.

If you don't hear or feel anything when you're listening, that is okay. Be patient. Be open. Be kind to yourself.

Connecting with the Soul and Something Greater Gives Comfort

Many patients I companioned at the ends of their lives felt connected to something greater. At this pinnacle of transformation, moving toward their death, they shifted out of their self-limiting thinking ego mind into their soul and felt an expansion and a vastness beyond. In their final days, these patients felt an undefinable timelessness and understood that their soul does not die. In this deep alignment with something greater, they felt vibrantly alive. When I saw them, their bodies and faces glowed.

One of these patients was Larry, an elderly man. In one of our visits, he told me that he'd had a near-death experience in his midthirties: During a routine surgery, he suddenly died. He remembered his soul leaving his body and walking down a long hallway, where he was greeted by a man in a long white robe. This man said to him, "It is not your time yet, Larry. You need to go back." Next thing Larry knew, he was seeing his body on the operating table, and then he was back in his body, lying on the table and hearing the voices of the operating-room technicians. Since that experience, he'd carried an understanding that death was not an end but a transformation.

Now, fifty years later, Larry was at the end of his life. In one of our last visits, he shared with me a dream he'd had the night before: "I traveled out of my body and looked down on myself lying in bed. A strong understanding came to me—it is now my time. And I am ready." He also knew deeply that he was not alone and was being held by something larger, which he called *God*. This knowledge was giving him comfort as he was getting ready to leave his body for good.

Larry was content and ready to go. He had no fear. He died peacefully two days after sharing his dream with me.

Not long after Larry's passing, I visited Sally, an elderly woman, a week before she died. "I dreamed that I died and saw the other side," she told me. "It was peaceful, and many of my deceased family members greeted me." She awakened in her bed feeling a deep knowing and trust. She, too, knew she was not alone and felt the peace of something larger, which she called *presence*, was with her and guiding her every step.

"I am ready. It is okay," she told me, squeezing my hand. A peace and warmth filled her entire bedroom.

Diane, another patient, was lying in bed, weak and in a contemplative mood, when I arrived for one of my last visits. Hearing that I was a chaplain, she told me, "I feel a strong presence, a force with me. I call it my higher power, and it is comforting." She also expressed a readiness to see what was next for her. I felt no fear present in the room—only peace was there. She died that weekend, peacefully, with a smile on her face.

Companioning hundreds of patients in their final days affirmed to me that each of us is a soul, in a body for a short time. Death is not an end. Our ego comes in at birth and dies at death, but our soul never dies. Our soul transforms into another form at the time of our death. There is also a force, something greater, that is present with us on every step of our life's path and beyond.

When we understand that there is something greater, that we are not alone, we can breathe more deeply, love more deeply, and feel more fully alive.

Connection Visualization

If you don't have a defined theology, belief, or name for something greater, you can still experience it. Even if you are not sure it exists, you can still experience it. Try this exercise and notice what you experience.

Become aware of any tension in your body and just breathe into that area for a moment. Breathe in peace; breathe out any stress that you may be holding.

Allow your mind and body to relax. Feel peace come through your body. If thoughts come into your mind, let them pass and go back to your breath—your in-breath, your out-breath.

You are relaxed.

Now imagine yourself in a beautiful meadow, surrounded by wildflowers. You can hear birds a little way off, and you know you are completely safe. You can feel the warmth of the sun on your face and body. As you gently lay down on the soft grass, feel the support of the earth and the warmth of the sun.

You are comfortable, relaxed, and safe. The earth is supporting your body.

Now visualize a golden light above your head. See it enter the top of your head. Flowing down through your head, neck, shoulders, and chest, it moves down through your entire body. It moves down through your stomach area, abdomen, into your legs, your knees, and down through your feet and out.

This light is cleansing, healing your body. Any tension and stress you may be holding is being released, and this light is healing and bathing your body as it moves through you.

Now focus on your heart. Invite it to soften. Feel your heart softening.

Bring to mind someone who is very easy for you to love. It could be a partner, child, parent, grandparent, friend, or pet. This person or animal may be living or dead. Whoever this being is, hold them in your heart. Allow yourself to feel warmth and love toward them. Notice how this warmth and love feels in your heart and in your body.

Breathe in love and breathe out love. Feel love expanding throughout your body and out around your body as you breathe. You are at peace.

Rest in this peace and love for the next few minutes.

We Are Not Alone: The Mystical Side of Connecting with Something Greater

Many mystics across all faith traditions have shared detailed accounts of their encounters with the unseen world. Throughout time, we hear of individuals touching into a realm that may not be perceived with the five physical senses. Their stories might seem extraordinary, but I can attest that when we connect with our souls and with something greater, it's possible we may open ourselves to what the mystics name and experience.

For me, the veil between this world and beyond opened not long after I'd left my corporate advertising job. I'd started doing some contract work with my husband's company. One day, while sitting in a conference room, listening to colleagues discuss marketing and web design, I looked up and was surprised to see dozens of pairs of eyes floating around the room. My colleagues were still there, seated around a large table. But between, around, and above them faint outlines of animal faces began to form. One of those closest to me looked like a wolf face.

Wow, what the . . . I thought. Then I felt an uncanny calmness come over me. I took a breath.

"Well, this is interesting," I said to myself. Somehow I was able to keep my composure, perhaps because I knew other people who'd had similar experiences.

After about ten minutes, the eyes disappeared. Though the meeting continued around me, I found myself distracted.

Afterward I started to regularly see sets of animal eyes and what looked like a wolf face floating around me. Fortunately, I had a mentor—a shamanic practitioner—who explained that what I'd seen were animal spirits. In many Native American spiritual traditions, the belief is that we all have animal spirits that guide us on our path. Michael helped me understand I was seeing totem animals, including my personal totem animal, a wolf. I learned that if I didn't want to see anything, I could say, "Stop, go away," and everything I was seeing with my intuitive sight would vanish.

Why I'd seen these animal spirits wasn't clear, but that first meeting with them was my introduction to a new way of seeing. I knew I had seen another dimension of reality. Because of my regular practices of coming into the present moment, connecting with my soul, and connecting with something greater, I was not distracted with my mind's myriad thoughts, but instead I was able to be fully present and open to the world around me, including the invisible layers. And I knew that what I'd seen was some sort of message from God.

After I became a chaplain, companioning so many people as they'd make the big leap to the other side gave me many opportunities to feel and experience the thin veil between us all. I often felt discernable shifts in the energy in patients' rooms when they died. Many patients' life energy grew larger, and I'd feel it move up through their body as their soul was about to leave. Their energy would then move up and out through their head as they took their last breath.

At night, at home in my bedroom, I would occasionally open my eyes to see a spirit hovering next to me or above me. I'd hear no words but see an outline of a human body, just clear enough for me to recognize the newly departed patient it belonged to. At first I'd gasp, feeling amazed and a bit taken aback. Then a strong feeling would come through me as the spirit of the patient said goodbye—and often thank you—before vanishing.

On one occasion, I was woken up by a large golden angel hovering over me. It then moved straight *into* my body. I felt a warmth and soothing feeling go through me, and I felt surprisingly calm and peaceful. I realized later that this angel was actually the guardian angel of a patient whom I'd been with as he died earlier that day, during my long night shift at a local trauma hospital. His angel had come to thank me.

These experiences confirmed my belief that death is a transformation, and we have many unseen guides, angels, and helpers with us along the way. They showed me how we are all interconnected to others through our souls and a felt sense of oneness and love, even after we die. I've found comfort in knowing we are not alone.

When I was companioning dying patients who had a sense of something more—their soul, an existence beyond physical death, and a felt sense of oneness with something greater—many of them also said they experienced, felt, sensed, or saw energy shifts and spirits from beyond.

My patient Ellen was just one example. During one of my visits, she told me that as a young girl she'd had a near-death experience while undergoing surgery. She'd seen her soul leaving her body and then found herself looking over her body on the operating table. She had seen and felt angels around her, and she knew that no matter what happened, she was going to be okay. That experience had been the beginning of her faith in God.

On the day she died, Ellen told me, "I saw my mother earlier this morning in the corner of the room, smiling at me. She is here. I am okay."

Ellen's mother had long been deceased. I could feel that we were not alone, and as I peered around the bedroom, I saw many spirits. Not only could I see their eyes and the outlines of their faces floating around Ellen's bed, but I also saw a warm, golden glow coming in through the window and surrounding her head. I know that feeling the presence of these spirits helped Ellen feel peace instead of fear when she died later that evening.

Another hospice patient, Diane, whom I introduced you to earlier in the chapter, also told me that she'd felt the spirits of loved ones: "Every night, in my dreams, my parents show up and tell me that they are waiting for me to come over." Stretched out in her dark bedroom, she said, "When I lay here in bed, I can feel their presence. I don't have any fear. I am looking forward to seeing them. I know I'm not alone."

Today I still see other dimensions of reality, and I'm grateful I'm allowed to see some of the layers that typically go unseen. I regard this ability as a gift, though it can have its challenges.

Once as I was reading a prayer at the bedside of a hospice patient, she gave a bloodcurdling growl, followed by a hiss. A pang of fear ran down my spine. I said a quick, silent prayer in my own mind, asking for love and light to surround me. Immediately I knew and felt I was protected and supported. At the end of the visit, as I was preparing to leave, I felt a sharp pain hit my neck, like something had tried to stab me. Afterward I realized the patient had been possessed by a negative entity, or "dark spirit." It had tried to attack me but had been thwarted by the force of love I'd called upon for protection.

This kind of negative encounter with spirits has been rare; I had only one other in my entire thirteen years as a chaplain. The more frequent challenge was receiving so many spirit visitors at night that I couldn't get enough sleep. I had to learn to put up energy boundaries: before I fell asleep, I'd say, "You cannot come within twenty feet of my bed while I'm sleeping." I also learned to be judicious about whose spirits I would invite to come and see me when they had passed. These measures cut down on my nightly spirit visitors dramatically.

I believe we all have intuitive gifts we can access safely and develop, if we choose. The ability to see different dimensions, for example, is an intuitive gift called *clairvoyance*. Some people see these dimensions in their mind's eye; others, like me, see them as if they were appearing before our physical eyes. Choosing to develop these spiritual gifts can often be a way of deepening our felt sense of interconnectedness and oneness with all and our connection to something greater.

You don't have to experience these mystical dimensions if you don't want to. You can experience awakening without seeing these other dimensions of reality. You can connect with your soul, with something greater, and with a felt sense of interconnectedness. You can take comfort in just knowing you are not alone in the universe—that there are unseen beings, spirits, with you. You don't have to label them or figure out their form and definition. You can just trust that there is something more. Opening to the spirit world and consciously inviting it in is another step. If you're interested, you might try my prayer: "Okay, God, lead me and guide me wherever you want me to go and see." Don't be disappointed if nothing happens, but don't be alarmed if it does.

Opening inward, feeling deeply, and touching into our soul, our essence, connects us with something greater. In this felt sense of oneness, of love, we may experience what is not visible to our eyes. I invite you to be open. No matter what, you will feel more alive and know you are not alone.

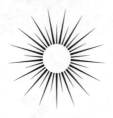

4

THE THIRD PRACTICE

Grow Your Trust

JACK WAS MY FIRST BOSS in the corporate advertising world back in the early nineties. A master salesman, gifted manager, and wonderful sales trainer, he one day left his successful advertising career after becoming disillusioned with the corporate world. Following a message from a still, small voice within, he packed up his bags and drove from Chicago to his hometown of St. Louis to stay with one of his brothers. Since then, he has picked up sporadic construction jobs that have helped him pay for his rent and food while he's dived deep into his spiritual practice.

Whenever I talk with him, he expresses no fear about his next paycheck, where he was going to land or live, or what his future holds. He exudes a calm confidence and a certainty that all is well. I always marvel at how he has been able to let go of the constant pressure to have a plan, a direction, and a defined purpose. Instead, he lives in the moment. He is able to take life as it unfolds, one day at a time, because he is living from a deep state of trust.

When I was a hospice chaplain, I regularly witnessed patients come to a similar deep state of trust. Facing their deaths, they turned inward and found a way to trust what was happening to them and how the ends of their lives were unfolding. Many patients moved from fearing death and the unknown to deeply trusting that they would be okay both while they were dying and after they had died.

The peace I tangibly felt with these patients, the peace I feel in Jack whenever I talk with him, is attainable now, for each one of us. The key to it lies in the third awakening practice: growing your trust.

The Practice of Trust

Trust is the practice of moving forward despite uncertainty, knowing that whatever happens, we can handle it. It doesn't mean doing something on impulse or acting without conscious thought and just hoping things will work out despite our fear. Instead, it means moving forward in vulnerability, knowing that we'll be okay despite that vulnerability. Many spiritual traditions call this faith. We may not have all the answers exactly when we want them, but we are open to whatever life is offering and how it is going. Trust enables us to move forward with the flow of life, as we will explore in the fifth awakening practice.

Trust starts with trusting ourselves—trusting our internal essence, our soul. We trust our inner voice, wisdom, and intuition—what some people might call our gut—instead of our fast-chattering ego mind. We feel rooted and grounded in something deep within ourselves rather than other people and other sources outside us.

For some of us, trust is also an outgrowth of our connection with something greater. Feeling the oneness that connects us all, we know we are not alone but are held and helped by something beyond us. We intentionally call upon it, lean into it, and find great comfort in knowing we are part of something greater than ourselves. Jack, for example, once shared with me, "I have never felt so alive and so connected to Source. Each day I let go and surrender my ego and trust." When I was going through cancer treatment as a child, I was able to trust that I would be okay because I felt I was connected to God. The same was true for many of the hospice patients I companioned. When we feel rooted and grounded in our connection with something greater, we develop a deep knowing that no matter what happens, "all shall be well and all manner of things shall be well," as the fourteenth-century mystic Julian of Norwich put it.

A lot of teachers and spiritual traditions talk about trust and why it is valuable. But too often trust is depicted as easy, as something we can one day just decide to do or an ability we can just turn on. If it were indeed easy, why do so many people struggle with it? The problem is, while a lot of sources talk about the importance of trust and encourage us to practice trust, very few actually teach us *how* to trust.

Fortunately, trust is something we can learn to do. I have found that trust rests on a foundation of *acceptance* and *deep listening*. Trust is almost impossible if we cannot do these two things, yet our trust will grow steadily if we practice accepting what is and listening deeply to our inner knowing.

What Is Your Relationship with Trust? (Part 1)

This journaling exercise invites you to consider what you currently think about the idea of trust.

Begin by sitting comfortably. Spend a few minutes focusing on your breath. Breathing in and breathing out, let your body relax and soften. Release any tension you may be holding in your body.

Now take a piece of paper or a journal and spend a few minutes on the following questions. Just write what comes to you, without censoring yourself.

> When was a time in your life that you felt trust? What did this trust look like? What did it feel like?
>
> What is your relationship with trust now?
>
> What keeps you from trusting now? What gets in the way?

When you're finished, just sit with what you wrote. Let go of any judgment that may arise and simply hold your answers.

We will come back to this journaling exercise at the end of the chapter.

Acceptance

Acceptance is seeing the moment for what it is, with no filter. We see things how they are, and instead of trying to change them, we choose to just be with them. We let go of the physical and mental energy of pushing and move into a space of neutrality. We let go of doing and move into being. We decide to stop trying to control, and we allow what is, the good and bad, to be just as it is.

Acceptance may include realizing there is a limit to what we can do to change something and stopping our efforts to do more than we can. Yet accepting things as they are doesn't mean pretending they are okay when they are not. It doesn't mean saying harm, abuse, or injustice, for example, are acceptable. Sometimes acceptance means acknowledging and facing difficult truths about what is. Sometimes it means acknowledging what needs to change.

Acceptance includes allowing any feelings we have about the present moment to be as they are. Instead of judging our feelings or trying to change them, we recognize them and allow them to be there as part of what is happening in the moment.

Acceptance also means allowing ourselves to be just the way we are in the moment. We don't suppress, reject, or deny who we are or any parts of who we are. We let go of our inner critic and self-judgment and accept ourselves fully. We also let others be who they are. We let go of our ego-based expectations of others, our attempts to get them to do what we want, and our judgments about what we think they should be doing or who we think they should be. Maybe we don't always agree with their behavior or choices, but we step back and let them live their lives and their truth. Accepting others is a first step in moving toward having love and compassion for others.

Practicing acceptance entails making a conscious internal shift. First, you recognize when your need to control has been activated. You notice the tight, grasping energy, and you name it. Just by acknowledging it, you can choose to accept it. And by accepting it, you can start to release the energy of control and its tight grip on you. You also feel any anger, frustration, or other feelings that are present, with no judgment. Finally, you accept and feel the uncertainty of the moment, again with no judgment. At first feeling the uncertainty may feel uncomfortable, because the ego mind likes to be in control. So you feel into that discomfort too. When you are able to let go of control and accept the uncertainty of the moment, you begin to open into the mystery of life.

Like being in the present moment, acceptance is a state we move in and out of throughout our daily lives. When we notice that we are resisting acceptance, we can pause and consciously decide to accept fully what is happening in the moment.

> *Whatever the present moment contains,*
> *accept it as if you had chosen it.*
> —Eckhart Tolle, The Power of Now

We suffer when, instead of accepting what is, we keep trying to control it. It is a natural human tendency to want to control as much as we possibly can. Acceptance can be very hard because our ego mind has strong ideas about how things should go. Underneath its attempts to maintain a grip on so much of life is fear. It is normal to fear the unknown, what the future holds, and something bad happening. But when our ego mind is running the show, we try to overcome our fear with grasping, clinging, and pushing. We create expectations about how things should be and should unfold. Then we feel anxious, disappointed, discouraged, demoralized, and more fearful when they don't go the way we planned. And even when things *do* go as we planned, we often feel empty, like something is missing. Our pushing and controlling behavior may satisfy our ego mind, but usually at the expense of us not feeling and not experiencing the wonder and mystery of life.

Many of us learn at an early age to try to control, shape, and mold every aspect of our lives. The fear-driven ego mind convinces us that striving and controlling are necessary for us to make our way in the world, and many people and other sources believe and reinforce this message. I certainly heard it growing up. I watched my entrepreneurial father, who ran several companies, push himself in his career, working very long hours, including weekends, in order to move out of his low-income childhood and into a "successful" life. He also pushed my siblings and me to work hard and strive to do our best. It was expected that we would get good grades in high school, go to a good college and excel there, and then, as my father would say, "be somebody in the world." His implicit message was that, to ensure our success, we had to control as much of our lives and our environment as possible.

Many people I have worked with over the years share his belief. Because of all their pushing and controlling, they have become high achievers—doctors, attorneys, business owners who have made their millions. They are also burned out. Or they feel empty, like something is missing. Either way, they are suffering physically, emotionally, and spiritually.

Ultimately, we learn that we simply cannot control every detail of our circumstances or all aspects of our lives, and trying to do so leads only to frustration, disappointment, discouragement, demoralization, anxiety, stress, and unrest.

Acceptance empowers us. It is often a relief to move out of the pushing, controlling energy of the ego mind and the suffering it creates. It is an act of self-love to let go of trying to control every aspect of ourselves, our circumstances, other people, or our lives all the time. Often, when we are able to accept what's happening, the good and the bad, there is an opening, an aha moment. The result is more freedom and more breathing room.

Like coming back to the present moment, acceptance is a skill you can learn. The more you practice it in small ways, the more you can do it when bigger situations arise. Driving in gridlock traffic, for example, is a great time to start practicing acceptance. The next time you're stuck in thick traffic, try noticing what is happening within you. You may notice your stress level increasing or a heat or tension rising in your body. You might notice feelings of angst, frustration, or irritation. In that moment, can you let go of trying to change the situation or wishing you could? Can you notice how you feel, without trying to change those feelings but without getting caught up in them either? Can you simply be in the present moment and accept what is happening within and around you, just as it is, in that moment?

> *True freedom is found in the absence of resistance.*
> —*Esther and Jerry Hicks,* Getting into the Vortex

Just because I know firsthand how valuable acceptance can be doesn't mean I always find it easy to do. When the coronavirus came to the United States in early 2020, my ability to accept uncertainty and things I couldn't change was severely tested. My husband, Scott, was on immunosuppressant drugs for his heart condition, so we needed to take extra precautions and avoid situations in which he might become ill. I struggled when I couldn't do so many of the little things I enjoyed, like meeting indoors with friends, going out to eat, and doing public speaking engagements in person. Our world became a small bubble indeed, and the changes we had to make—big and small—were hard for me to make peace with, especially when I saw friends and neighbors whose lives never changed.

Meanwhile, in some of my meditation practices, when I was very still, I'd feel the upheaval and anguish in the world, along with all the illness and death, and I'd break down crying. How could I just accept that so many people were being hospitalized and dying? How was I supposed to accept not knowing when or if this pandemic was going to end? Finally, I realized I had to accept what was happening—to me, to my family, to the world. Choosing to accept this new reality, as well as how I felt about it, was the first necessary step. From that place of acceptance, I could choose how to live.

Every day we are consciously choosing to practice acceptance, or we are subconsciously choosing to hold tight to how we want things in our lives to unfold and our attempts to control each step. When we accept what is, we let go of the illusion that we're actually in control, and we open the door for allowing things to unfold according to their own flow. We can then live with a heightened sense of presence, accepting the moment and opening into the mystery and flow of life.

When we practice acceptance, our energy flows more freely and is more assessable to us because it is not tied up with and consumed by trying to create a certain outcome. There is more breathing room and space for us to be present and open into the unlimited possibilities. And when we can feel those possibilities, our ability to trust that we are being guided on our path grows.

> *Whatever happens. Whatever what is is is*
> *what I want. Only that. But that.*
> —*Galway Kinnell, "Prayer"*

Just Let It Be

The following exercise will help you come into the present moment and notice what acceptance feels like.

Take a minute and let your body relax. Drop your shoulders and focus on your breath, breathing in and breathing out.

Notice whatever is present in your body right now. If you are feeling unrest, tightness, or pain, physical or emotional, in your body, just breathe into that area.

As you breathe into this area of your body, notice what is there. No need to change, judge, or analyze anything. Just breathe and feel.

Stay with any physical sensation and feel it in your body. Notice whatever is present.

Accept this moment as is.

Let whatever is there be there as you continue breathing in and out for a couple of minutes.

Now take a moment and notice how you feel after accepting what you are feeling. Is the pain, tightness, unrest you felt in your body still there? Has it loosened, shifted, softened, or otherwise changed in any way? It is fine if it didn't. Just continue to notice what is present and continue breathing in and out.

Spend the next few minutes breathing in and out. Being present with whatever arises.

Spiritual Acceptance

Spiritual traditions over the ages have talked about acceptance as surrendering to something greater than ourselves. To me, this means surrendering the will of our ego mind to a greater or higher power. Personally, I find great comfort in this idea, and many of my clients do too. For other clients, spiritual acceptance takes the form of surrendering the will of their ego mind to what their internal wisdom, their true nature, wants for them.

I see spiritual acceptance as a way of opening to an unlimited universal energy. I believe this energy is both within us (imminent) and outside us (transcendent), and it is accessible to all of us when we can accept what is present for us in this moment. When we don't accept what is, we deny how this greater energy is moving within and around us. Our life becomes tight, controlled, and lacking aliveness because we are living out of only our ego mind and not our whole being, which is connected to an even greater whole.

Accepting the uncertainty of the moment is another aspect of spiritual acceptance. It could be also referred to as "living in the unknown" or "opening into the mystery." It is in this liminal space of the unknown, the mystery, that we can feel the magic, magnetic, electric energy of life.

Finally, I believe spiritual acceptance includes accepting our limitations, disappointments, unmet expectations, pain, and even death as parts of our lives. By accepting all of life, we find new life. We open into and feel the energy of life moving within us. This energy, this force, empowers us and expands our view of what can be possible beyond the limits of our ego mind.

When we surrender our ego mind to the will of a greater force, we create space for freedom to enter. We let go and feel into the unlimited possibilities and then have room to trust more.

Be nothing, do nothing, get nothing, become nothing,
seek for nothing, relinquish nothing.
—Miranda Macpherson, The Way of Grace

Acceptance Meditation 1

Like the earlier exercise "Just Let It Be," this guided meditation will allow you to experience acceptance.

Take the next five minutes to come into the present moment. Feel into your heart area and just breathe. Accept and surrender any attachments in the moment. Let go and accept the moment completely, just as it is.

Tune in to what comes to you as you're accepting. What is here? What do you feel? What do you notice? Can you feel energy moving in your body within and/or outside your body? What are you noticing and feeling in your body and in your heart right now?

The felt sense of acceptance feels different for all of us, and each person will describe it differently. For me, it feels like a soothing energy moving up and down my body, along with an emerging sense of connectedness and oneness. One of my clients says acceptance feels grounding and centering to her. Another client says she feels that a force, a strength, something beyond her, is holding her. Others find it impossible to express in words the way acceptance feels and instead use drawing, painting, or movement, such as dance.

What does acceptance feel like for you? And how can you best express that feeling?

If it feels right, take a minute and write down a few notes about what you experienced during this meditation. That way, you can come back and try it again and see what else surfaces.

Calming Our Nervous System Helps Us Practice Acceptance

Acceptance is often not easy, for several good reasons. Life can be hard and challenging, and we often have to endure unwelcome changes, upheaval, loss, and harm. The ego mind and our fear-feeding culture only add to our ongoing stress. When we are in a state of stress, our nervous system can easily become dysregulated, making it difficult for us to accept what's happening in the present moment without trying to change or control it.

Our nervous system moves naturally through three states in daily life. The parasympathetic state—where we feel safe, calm, grounded, and connected to those around us—is meant to be our baseline. From there, we will move into one of the other two states: a mobilized fight-or-flight state or an immobilized freeze state. When we work out, for example, we will move into a mildly mobilized (fight-or-flight) state, and when we sleep, we move into a mildly immobilized (freeze) state. We are meant to move into a heightened fight-or-flight or a freeze state during serious life stresses or when we're threatened, in order to escape or survive danger. In an ideal world, we would move into the most intense versions of the fight-or-flight and freeze states only briefly. Once the stress or threat has been addressed, and we know we are safe again, we would easily return to our baseline parasympathetic state. But the world is not always ideal. Things like past trauma, ongoing stress, or a lengthy challenging situation can keep us in a heightened fight-or-flight or freeze state for so long that this state becomes our new baseline.

Whenever we're in a heightened fight-or-flight or freeze state, we may experience symptoms of nervous system dysregulation. Physically, our heartbeat and breathing may become erratic. We may experience shortness of breath, nausea or stomach upset, or irritable bowels. Mentally, we may have difficulty focusing. Emotionally, we may experience anxiety, depression, panic, or numbness. These symptoms dissipate usually naturally after the highly stressful or emergency situation has passed and we've shifted back to our parasympathetic baseline. But when we've stayed in a heightened fight-or-flight or freeze state so long that it has become our new normal, these symptoms of dysregulation tend to become chronic problems.

Learning to calm our nervous system and return to a parasympathetic state after being in a dysregulated state is important for our long-term health and well-being. And it is often a necessary first step if we want to practice acceptance.

As I shared in chapter 1, Scott was once hospitalized for a very serious cardiac condition. A few days into his hospital stay, my son and I left the hospital to pick up some food. While we were at the local grocery store, I got a phone call from the cardiologist. Scott's heart rate was dropping, and he needed to have an external pacemaker put in to keep his heart going. We rushed back to the hospital just in time to see him being wheeled into surgery.

What is happening? I thought. *Is he going to live?*

I began pacing the floor. I felt panic rising in my chest. I wanted to scream.

Stepping onto an outdoor patio, I called my close friend Laurie. She immediately said, "Stop. I am here with you. Go sit or lay down. Let's breathe together."

I lay down on a bench, and with her guidance, I took several deep breaths into my abdomen. As I kept breathing deeply, my heart rate slowed, and my nervous system gradually shifted out of the overwhelming fight-or-flight state. My stress level dropped, and some space started to enter my body. Once I was back in a parasympathetic state, I was able to come back to the present moment and accept what was happening.

The deep belly breathing Laurie had prompted me to do had calmed my mobilized nervous system by stimulating my vagus nerve. Also known as the tenth cranial nerve, the vagus nerve connects our brain to our gut and communicates messages to our central nervous system. Activating or stimulating our vagus nerve through deep abdominal breathing moves us back into a calm, parasympathetic state.

There are many other ways we can calm our dysregulated nervous system during overwhelmingly stressful times. The three exercises at the end of this section offer more options for you to experiment with. They will not only help you during stressful situations; doing these exercises on a daily basis can also help your nervous system learn to regulate itself more easily.

In addition to calming your nervous system, learning how to safely feel your feelings and release blocked, trapped, or stifled emotions, as described in chapter 2's exercise "Retrain Your Negative-Thinking Mind," will also support your ability to practice acceptance.

Please note: The long-lasting effects of trauma on the nervous system can make it especially difficult to practice acceptance and therefore to grow your trust. If you have experienced trauma, working with a trauma-informed mental health professional can be helpful. Sometimes practicing acceptance means accepting that we cannot do something on our own and we need support and guidance.

Tapping to Calm Yourself

The Emotional Freedom Technique (EFT), also known as tapping, is a practice in which you tap on acupressure points to help calm and balance the energy in your body. Tapping can help release emotional and physical pain and discomfort. It can also help you regulate your nervous system state in times of stress.

With this exercise, you will calm your nervous system by tapping an acupressure point on your hand known as the gamut point. This spot is located on the back of your hand between the bones of your last two fingers (your ring finger and little finger), midway between your knuckles and your wrist. All you need to do is use the fingers of your opposite hand to tap on this gamut point for a few minutes.

If after a few minutes you still feel stressed, you can tap on another acupressure point found under either eye, in the middle of your lower eye bone. Tap on this second point for another minute or so.

You do not need to say any words as you tap. Just feel your feelings of stress and unrest as you continue tapping and breathing. Keep tapping and breathing into the feelings until you feel calmer.

Alternate Shoulder Tapping

This exercise uses a different kind of tapping to calm your nervous system. It is helpful in both stressful situations and for chronic stress.

Cross your arms over your chest so your hands rest on the opposite shoulders—right hand on left shoulder, left hand on right shoulder. Start alternately tapping your hands on your shoulders. Just breathe regularly as you continue tapping for ten minutes. Then stop and notice how you feel when you have finished.

If you have chronic stress, you can use this exercise daily. Try doing it five times a day, for ten minutes each time, for seven days. At the end of the seven days, notice whether you feel calmer and more relaxed during the day.

OM Toning

This exercise will not only help stimulate your vagus nerve and tell your body to relax but will also help you come back to the present moment.

Sit or stand comfortably. Focus on your breath, breathing in and out, for a few moments.

Now take a deep breath in, and on the out breath, sound the word *om* (pronounced with a long *o* sound, like in the word *home*). Continue sounding *om* until you need to take a breath in.

Take another breath, and then on your out breath, sound *om* again.

Repeat this pattern for the next minute, feeling what is present in your body as you tone the word *om*. Where you able to feel the energy moving in your body? What does this energy feel like?

After toning *om* for one minute, stop and resume breathing naturally. How do you feel?

The word *om* is actually a letter from ancient Sanskrit (circa 1500–1200 BCE). Found in the Upanishads, *om* is also a sacred word referring to "the mystery." It has been referred to as the ancient sound for life and all creation. It is a powerful word historically used in mantras, chanting, and yoga practices to promote harmony and oneness with universal energy.

Acceptance Opens the Door for Change

David had a successful personal training business and competed in national bodybuilding competitions. One day he pulled a muscle in his knee. He tried to power forward, but instead of healing, his knee only became more painful, tight, and stiff. Over the course of several months, the pain became so much worse that he had to cut back the number of clients he saw and miss the competitions he had planned on attending. Shaken to the core, he became consumed with thoughts about both the pain and how it was interfering with his daily life and work.

Late one afternoon, while sitting in a hot tub at the local YMCA, David felt all the tension and stress running through his body. He'd hit a wall. He realized his negative-thinking mind and fearful thoughts were stifling him. In that moment, he surrendered.

"I fully accepted that I may not be able to compete again," he told me. "I said to the universe, 'If this is how my knee is going to be, I surrender. Help me. And if there can be healing, let it be so.' I then let go of my fear and negative thoughts and accepted completely what was happening."

At that moment, as David accepted his situation, his body relaxed. All his contracted muscles let go, softened, and lengthened, and there was a notable energy shift and release in the area. The pain and tightness in his knee disappeared, and he had full movement in the joint again.

At the same time, he heard the words, "I am with you." Tears came to his eyes.

Our mind, body, and spirit are all connected. David's healing happened when he realized his fearful negative thoughts were making his physical problem worse, and he let them go and accepted what was happening to him.

It may seem like a paradox, but accepting what's happening without trying to change it is often what allows change to happen. Acceptance doesn't guarantee that things will be fine or circumstances will shift, but it can open the door for change.

Acceptance Meditation 2

In this guided meditation, we will stop resisting, fighting, and judging what is happening in this moment and practice accepting this moment just as it is.

I invite you to close your eyes. Bring your attention to your breath, breathing in and breathing out.

Become aware of any tension in your body. Just breathe into that tense area for a moment.

Notice any thoughts that arise. See them like clouds in the sky, coming and going.

You are the vast, blue, endless sky that is unchanging. Any thoughts that arise just float up and out and pass by.

If any emotions surface, don't resist or fight them. Just feel and experience them.

Emotions are not permanent. When we feel our feelings, they start to open and move through us. If fear, anxiety, or unrest arise, let yourself be with them, feel them, and they will move through you.

Then there will be room for love, light, and peace to come in.

Just let yourself be.

You are here, now, alive.

Feel your heart beating.

Feel your body expand as your breath comes in and then recede as your breath goes out.

Accept this moment fully.

Accept what is, as it is.

Continue breathing in and breathing out.

Now put your hands over your heart area. Our bodies always respond to physical touch. Notice how your body starts to soften and relax.

Feel your heart soften and expand.

You might say to yourself, "May I be at peace."

Feel peace in your heart.

Continue breathing in and breathing out for the next few minutes.

When you are ready, you can gently open your eyes.

Practicing Acceptance at the End of Life

Upon my first visit with Rebecca, the energy in her bedroom was tense. She tried to smile, but she looked exhausted and depleted. She talked about how she hoped to get stronger and be able to start another cancer treatment.

Forty-five-year-old Rebecca had been a successful executive, a mother, a spouse, and an athlete who had many friends and was well loved. She had a dazzling smile and beauty about her. After being diagnosed with a rare form of cancer, she aligned with the motto "I will fight, and I will survive." She researched every medical treatment available in the country. When possible, she would try a new clinical trial yearly. During five long years of treatments, she had been able to keep working part time and enjoy family and friends. But the cancer remained, despite all the treatments, and the doctors had recently told Rebecca no other options were available.

Still, Rebecca held out hope for another possible treatment. She tried to exert her control, and she continually played through various scenarios about what medical center she could go to next and what new treatment option she could possibly qualify for. Meanwhile, however, her blood levels kept dropping, and she needed weekly blood transfusions to keep her body stable.

She was not willing to accept what was happening. Instead, she was grasping and clinging to what she wanted to happen. Fear was running through her, and her mind was running what little remained of her life. It was impossible for her to take in the preciousness of moments with her family because she was focused only on fighting every step of her path.

Rebecca's fight to live, to push away death, was actually causing her more suffering. Her will, her fighting, her pushing created an air of unrest that was palpable within her and around her. Watching her decline, her nonacceptance, and her push to stay alive took its toll on her family.

A week after I met her, Rebecca had trouble getting out of bed and reluctantly entered hospice. Her comments told me that she was continuing to strive to control what was happening. Within a few days, however, she started to transition—the phase that comes before someone moves into actively dying—and she was coming in and out of consciousness.

Two days later I sat on Rebecca's bed next to her. I could feel that she had made a palpable shift. When we talked about what she loved, she named her family and husband. A smile came over her face, and tears welled up in her eyes. Words were few between us. I held her hand as she gently opened and closed her eyes.

Rebecca had surrendered, had let go of her tight grip and control, and accepted the reality of what was happening. She was calm. A softening and ease moved within and around her.

We sat together in stillness until a few family members came in. Then Rebecca's eyes opened wide. She became more alert and thanked her mother and sister for who they were in her life. A peace and warmth filled the room as we all sat together, and her family shared stories, laughter, and tears. An ease and stillness lingered in the room as I left.

Rebecca had moved from pushing to accepting and trusting how the last hours of her life were unfolding. She died in the middle of the night.

Acceptance can give us a lot of relief and new life. When we push and control, we expend a lot of life energy, and we often miss out on the beauty of what is present and what it means to be alive right now. The day before she died, Rebecca finally felt relief and peace when she accepted what was happening. This peace helped her let go.

Rebecca showed me how trying to control what's happening instead of accepting it can cause us more pain and suffering. Another hospice patient, Sue, decided early on that she was going to accept what was happening to her, and she had a very different experience.

I met sixty-five-year-old Sue a day after she entered hospice. She had been dealing with a rare heart condition for the last seven years, and she explained that on the day she learned of it, she'd decided to embrace life.

"I decided I wanted to learn and grow until the day I died," she shared. "I want to live and open, not shut down. I want to live in the mystery."

As we sat together in her living-room area, she told me of what she had learned over the past seven years. "I understand what it means to love—to really feel love in my heart. I have never felt so alive as I have this past year," she said.

She shared a number of recent experiences she'd had with her family and friends and talked about the wonder of life all around her. I marveled at how she had accepted her health condition and at her determination to feel every drop of life, even as she expressed curiosity about what was on the other side of it.

Two weeks later, when she was near death, I was called in to see her. A warmth and a felt sense of presence and ease drafted through her bedroom. I offered prayers of thanksgiving for her life and our friendship and well-wishes for her transition over to the other side. She passed late that night with a smile on her face.

Sue experienced new life in the last year as she accepted her health condition and trusted the next steps on her path. This acceptance allowed her to open fully, feel, and grow until the last day of her life.

The message here is not to give up and not fight when facing extraordinary challenges but to find the balance between moving forward and doing what we can and accepting what we cannot do. Not being able to accept what is happening only causes us more undue stress and suffering. But practicing acceptance allows us to trust whatever may come and to live more fully, even at the end of life.

Deep Listening

When we can fully accept each moment exactly as it is, we open the door for deep listening.

When I told my father I planned to go to graduate school, he was appalled. "You want to study geology?" he yelled incredulously.

"No, *theology*," I corrected.

He didn't like this answer any better and continued to yell about what a big mistake I was making. Neither his opposition nor the lukewarm response from other family members bothered me though. Even though I didn't know exactly where my path was heading, a feeling inside me told me studying theology was the next step for me, and I trusted that inner knowing.

This inner knowing hadn't developed overnight. It was the culmination of several months of deep inner listening. When I had quit my job at Time Warner, I didn't know what the next steps on my path would be, but I knew I'd be able to discern them if I took time to listen to my heart and soul. So I had devoted time every day to meditating, walking, and journaling. I carved out times to just breathe, to practice presence, and to experience space and stillness. I purposely created the conditions for receiving wisdom and guidance from within and from my connection with something greater.

Deep listening means intentionally setting yourself up to receive inner guidance or answers when you have a specific question or concern. It can also mean just paying attention and staying open to general guidance from within during your daily life. In both cases, you are tuning in to and noticing the many ways you can hear, sense, and feel information coming to you from beyond the limited view of the ego mind.

The first step is carving out time when you tune out the noise of the outer world and tune in to how you feel internally. If you find it hard to slow down your mind, start small. Practice just coming back to the present moment, which will quiet your mind and allow you to feel some inner spaciousness. You could also meditate or practice yoga. Take a walk outside or spend time in nature. Relax in a hot bath. Do some journaling to help you process what is moving in your mind.

The next step is asking for help from your soul and the universal life energy it's connecting you to. These sources of wisdom are always present and guiding your life. The more you turn inward and pay attention to them, the more you can hear, feel, and discern the movement and guidance of these sources of your inner wisdom.

When you are listening deeply, you can hear, in small moments, the many messages that are available to you daily. These messages may arise directly from your inner wisdom in the form of feelings, sensations, nudgings, or knowings. A sensation in your body might draw your attention to a particular person or situation. An emotion might contain healing information from your soul. These internal messages may come to you during the times you specifically dedicate to deep listening, such as when you're journaling, meditating, or practicing presence. They may also arise spontaneously as you're going about your daily life, and you will easily recognize them because you have taken the time to establish the connection with your inner wisdom.

Your inner voice may also speak to you through external sources. Messages may come in the form of signs—things you see or notice in daily life that your inner wisdom says are more meaningful than just coincidences. Messages may come through other people: In a conversation with friends, one of them unwittingly says something that speaks directly to the topic you're seeking guidance about. Or a chance encounter with an old acquaintance or a neighbor leads you to exactly the person who can help you. Or something you randomly read at the checkout counter at the grocery store, hear on the radio in the car, or see on TV triggers an inner aha moment.

Deep listening doesn't necessarily mean the answers and guidance you're seeking will come right away. You may need to practice accepting uncertainty and feeling whatever emotions arise as you're waiting, such as fear, anxiety, irritation, and impatience. If you are not in a state of acceptance, you are putting conditions on the messages and guidance you want to receive. You're asking to hear what you want to hear, and perhaps also when and how you want to hear it, instead of being willing to accept whatever your inner wisdom and the flow of life have to say. Personally, I have found that the more I practice accepting the uncertainty and uncomfortable energy of the moment, the more I can hear. Otherwise, my mind tends to spin off into stress and anxiety, overwhelming my inner voice.

Just because you are deeply listening for guidance doesn't mean you will get the answers you want. It can sometimes be challenging to accept the messages you receive. I learned this lesson firsthand even before I left my advertising job at Time Warner. I had been offered a management job—a job I had asked for and even written the job description for. Yet when it came time for me to accept the position, the word *yes* would not come out of my mouth. Instead, a deep inner feeling said no. I spent the entire weekend crying because I didn't know what to make of this message. How could my corporate career be coming to an end? And if it was, why didn't I know where I was being led next?

I had a similar experience a few years later after I finished graduate school, when I decided to explore chaplain training. I'd looked into all the chaplain residency programs in the Twin Cities and was fortunate to be accepted into those offered by all the major hospital systems. When I prayed about what program to choose, I kept feeling a nudging to go to the one at the University of Minnesota—the very hospital where I'd spent years going through intensive treatment as a child. This was *not* the guidance I wanted. Unrest and anxiety ran through my body at the thought, and I dismissed the idea. But finally, a month later, I leaned into this deep-felt guidance, swallowed a courage pill, and started chaplain training at the university hospital. During that time, I experienced a new, deeper level of healing around my childhood experience there. Clearly, my soul had guided me back to the hospital where I had been a patient for more than just professional reasons.

Deep listening can help us not only when we're facing big decisions but also in our day-to-day activities. After I became a chaplain, my regular practice of deep listening helped me hear useful messages as I worked overnight on-call shifts for our local trauma hospital. When I left the hospital at 4:00 a.m., tired and emotionally drained, I would pray, "Okay, I have had enough. Please let me be done for the night."

Sometimes I'd hear my inner guidance reply, "You are done." Other times I'd hear, "One more page," and I'd know I had to prepare myself. No matter what message I heard, this inner guidance always comforted me. I knew I was not alone but had help from spiritual sources as I was doing my chaplain work.

Today I am still guided by my inner wisdom. I have learned over the years that it's easier to hear its guidance when I am still, present, and silent. I set aside time to meditate and walk, or journal, every day. Asking for guidance and listening for answers and words of insight is a normal part of my daily life.

I believe we all have the capacity for deep listening and receiving guidance from our soul and the ever-present universal energy that connects us all. Hearing this guidance may take practice, but it is here and waiting within each of us to be discovered.

The more you listen deeply, the more you will open into and hear the guidance that is within and all around you. The more you listen inwardly, even for a few small moments at a time, the more your intuition, your deep inner knowing, surfaces, and the more conscious you become. You begin to see with the eye of your soul. You will begin to trust that life and your path are unfolding exactly as they are meant to.

What Is Life Giving? A Deep Listening Exercise

This is one of my favorite exercises. I have practiced it for over twenty years. It comes from the spiritual exercises of Saint Ignatius of Loyola. It's an example of one way we can listen to our soul and open to its guidance on a daily basis.

At the end of each day, ask yourself the following two questions and then listen deeply for answers:

> What today has been life giving?
> What today has depleted you, drained you, taken life away?

From a Christian perspective, "life giving" means supporting "the fruits of the spirit"—peace, joy, love, how God is moving and leading you. From an ecumenical perspective, it means what has made you feel good and uplifted.

You might start a journal in which you answer these two questions every day over a few weeks. If you do, you will likely start to see patterns. You'll see what people, experiences, events, and situations are consistently lifting you up and which are not.

Listening Deeply in Stressful Moments

As I was driving to see my father in his final days in hospice, I found myself pleading to God, "Help me, guide me, fill me with your love and light! This is hard!" Then I accepted and opened into the mystery of what was going to happen.

I heard a voice in my mind say to me, "He is going to die today."

This message from my inner guidance confirmed my feeling that I had only a few precious moments left with my father.

I know I could not have heard my inner voice speak to me so clearly that morning if I had not already been practicing deep listening so regularly that it had become second nature. Listening deeply can be very hard when we are under great stress. During these times, we often can't get out of our busy mind, and our nervous system can easily become dysregulated. It can be virtually impossible to hear our internal wisdom and its guidance under these conditions. I also want to acknowledge that listening to our internal wisdom, feelings, and guidance can be challenging at any time if in the past we have experienced trauma or upheaval during which we felt no inner guidance or even felt we had been misguided.

Laying the foundations for deep listening during less stressful times makes it more likely we will be able to stay in touch with our inner wisdom in stressful situations. Through the first awakening practice, coming back to the present moment, we establish the habit of quieting our minds, feeling our feelings, and creating inner stillness and silence. Through the second awakening practice, connecting to something greater, we grow accustomed to touching into our soul, the source of our inner wisdom, and feeling the universal energy or life force that is available to us all.

From there, we practice accepting what the present moment is offering, whatever it is, exactly as it is, without judgment. Then we take time to regularly unplug from external and internal distractions and then tune in to our inner wisdom, and the something greater it's connected to. Doing all these things again and again as we move through the typical ups and downs of our daily lives will help us stay connected to and hear our inner voice no matter what is happening around us.

I also make sure to soothe my nervous system on a regular basis, using techniques like those in the exercises earlier in this chapter. Using those calming techniques daily helps keep my nervous system from becoming dysregulated when I'm under stress. Using them in overwhelming moments brings me back to a regulated, parasympathetic state, where I'm able to once again accept what is happening in the present moment, reconnect with God and my inner wisdom, and open again to hearing their guidance.

Like the first two awakening practices, listening deeply becomes easier to do the more you practice. The more you practice listening to your inner wisdom, the easier it will be able to stay open to hearing it when you need its guidance the most.

Everyday Trust

The more we practice acceptance, and the more we listen for and follow our inner guidance, the more we learn to trust ourselves and trust life. For me, trust has been instrumental to awakening and living fully. It is what has allowed me to move forward in my life even amid the unknowns.

When my friend suggested I attend graduate school to study theology, a strong feeling within confirmed this was the next step on my path. I trusted this gut feeling, and I moved forward despite the uncertainty of not knowing what the step after that might be. Similarly, when I started my first chaplaincy position at a long-term specialty care facility, I trusted it was the next step on my path even though I didn't know where this path was going.

This specialty care center focused on complex chronically ill patients. The first month I worked there, I took my lunch breaks in an eighth-floor conference room. I'd sit and eat my lunch by myself, looking out the windows over the Minneapolis skyline, and see the building where, only a few years prior, I had been working as a senior media executive. That job had been glamorous; I made great money and had a big expense account, a secretary, and a company car. Now I was sitting in a medical center conference room on my own, reviewing the challenging patients I saw that morning and the grave illnesses and suffering I had witnessed. I gazed out at the skyline and felt confused. *What am I doing with my life? Who am I now?* I thought.

I accepted and lived in this uncomfortable feeling for weeks. Amid the many daily questions from my ego mind and the continual feeling of unease and loneliness, I leaned into the knowing within that confirmed I was in the right place. Listening to that knowing, I trusted and moved forward. I took a deep breath and continued trusting my decision to work at this center each day. As the next month rolled in, I started to feel and understand how this new path suited me, and I started to love my chaplaincy work.

Our trust grows when we practice accepting the moment for what it is, even if it is uncomfortable. Our trust grows when we learn to tune in to what our soul and our inner wisdom are telling us. Our inner knowing comes through when we are living in the present moment, accepting what is, and listening deeply. And when we accept and embrace what arises—what we hear, sense, or feel beyond our ego mind—we can move forward, knowing and trusting we are being guided along our path.

The more we grow our trust, the more peace and equanimity we will feel. We begin to understand that we are here on this earth for a reason. Instead of worrying about what will happen next, we start trusting our path as it unfolds. We can be in the here and now. We can feel fully alive.

What Is Your Relationship with Trust? (Part 2)

Now that you have explored and practiced acceptance and deep listening, it's time to reconsider your relationship with trust. In a journal or on a new sheet of paper, answer these questions:

> How do you feel about trust now?
> Does trust feel any more available to you now? How much?

Write whatever comes to you, with no judgment.

When you are done writing, notice if your answers changed since you moved through this chapter and its exercises.

A Prayer for Growing Your Trust

Here is a prayer you can say silently or out loud to support the growth of trust:

> *May I trust and accept what is, right now, despite my uncertainty.*
> *May I listen within to hear the movement of my soul.*
> *May I feel strength as I move forward.*
> *Help me to trust.*
> *Help me to feel my light within and around me in this moment.*
> *I let go.*
> *I surrender.*
> *I trust.*

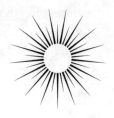

5

THE FOURTH PRACTICE

Embody Love

DRIVING UP TO THE AIRPORT, I see my friend Laurie standing at the end of the passenger platform, waving at me with a big smile. I pull up, and she jumps in my car and gives me a hug.

"Hello, my dear," she says. Her warmth, love, and big energy fill my entire car.

Later that afternoon, as she and I go for a walk, Laurie is smiling, greeting many people, and talking to every dog that passes by. People tend to gravitate toward her, and I can feel them softening and opening as she connects with them. I marvel at how she is so open and accepting of everyone.

"When I share my love, I feel more love, and feel fully alive," Laurie has told me.

To me, Laurie is a living example of embodied love. She feels so much love in her being that everyone around her can feel it in their own bodies. In her presence, I feel more alive and a stronger sense of love and oneness with all.

I believe embodying love is essential to awakening. If you can't feel the warm sensation of love in your heart and body, you cannot feel fully alive. The more you feel love, the more it flows throughout your whole being, and the more alive you feel. The more we embody love, the more we open into and grow the love that we are.

When I was a hospice chaplain, love was the number-one theme I heard people talk about on their deathbed. Hundreds of people at the end of their life told me that all they wanted was love—to deeply feel and be love. Everything else had dropped away. They were able to let go of their angst and grudges and find openness, space, and ease. I saw many of these people open to and fully embody love. Some had notable physical healings as a result; others healed emotionally and spiritually. Many had a glow about them and radiated a transcendent, otherworldly peace. For many of them, feeling this much love in their being was an aha moment. "Oh, so this is why I am here on this earth," they would say in wonder.

I experienced the power of embodied love when my husband was in the hospital, and we didn't know whether he would live or die. Despite my anxiety, I felt love in my body and being at a depth I had never before. Afterward I decided I wanted to continue feeling that way because the more I did, the more vibrantly alive I felt.

When we don't embody love, we miss out on the warmth and healing energy of love. People often struggle to embody love because they hold only a mental understanding of love. We can't feel love in our minds. Living solely in our mind keeps us from feeling love in our heart, body, and being.

There are several reasons we may only think about love instead of feeling it. Perhaps we grew up not feeling loved. We may not have received love from and formed healthy connections and attachments with our parents or caregivers, family members, or other loved ones in our early childhood. Maybe we have been hurt, abandoned, or never experienced unconditional love. Maybe we have grown up shutting down or blocking our emotions. Whatever the reason, too many of us don't really know what love actually feels like, much less how to embody it.

The first three awakening practices have already helped you open the door to embodying love. In addition, practicing self-love, forgiveness, gratitude, and sharing love with others; remembering times we have given or received deep love; getting out of the habit of judging others; and releasing buried and blocked emotions are ways we can support our ability to embody more and more love.

Self-Love

In my thirties, I found myself at a turning point where I wanted to feel more self-love. Growing up in a household where we didn't talk about feelings, I was ready to feel more love in my body. I thought that if I could feel more self-love, my heart would open and grow. If I felt more love, I'd have more love to share with my family and friends.

I engaged in a practice called mirror work, which I learned from the late Louise Hay, who greatly influenced my life at that time. Mirror work entails looking intently into your eyes in the mirror and telling yourself "I love you" repeatedly for a few minutes. I practiced this mirror work every day for a month. At the end of the month, as I looked into my eyes, I saw a softening. I felt a distinct sensation, a flutter and deepening, in my heart area. I felt more self-love, and my heart felt larger and fuller.

Feeling this love in my heart throughout the day, I was able to more clearly notice when I would get caught up in my thinking mind and was not feeling my feelings.

> *Love yourself as much as you can, and all of*
> *life will mirror this love back to you.*
> —Louise Hay, You Can Heal Your Life

Loving yourself is critical to embodying love. I believe we can't fully embody love if we don't love ourselves. Without self-love, there is a vacancy, a hole, an emptiness that keeps us from experiencing the full embodiment of love. Self-love is not selfish; it is essential to feeling fully alive and being able to love others. We can't fully give to another without loving ourselves.

If we want to embody love, we need to remove the barriers that keep us from feeling love for ourselves.

Feeling self-love is hard for many people. It may seem like a foreign and unattainable concept if our family of origin didn't support and encourage feeling love for ourselves, or if our personal history includes trauma or chronic fear and anxiety. A lack of self-love doesn't mean you are unlovable or that something is wrong with you. I believe anyone who wants to feel more love for themselves can learn to do so. Growing your self-love is a practice.

In one of my first visits with Marcia, she said she didn't feel love for herself or feel like she had much love to give to others. She had grown up in a home where the messages she heard were negative, critical, and unsupportive. Her mother was narcissistic, and most of her childhood memories consisted of her supporting her mother. As she and I unpacked her childhood, we explored attachment theory, which looks at how our connection with our primary caregiver in early childhood shapes our emotional and social development and ability to connect with others. Marcia was able to grieve for the love she had not received as a child, including a warm, loving relationship with her main caregivers. I then introduced the power of self-love, and we explored several practices to help her develop love for herself, including the meditation at the end of this section.

A month later, Marcia shared, "I'm finally feeling love in my heart. I'm feeling a sense of aliveness that I've never felt before! I am committed to practicing self-love every day. I notice that when I do I have more love to share with my kids and my husband."

Loving ourselves means caring for our physical, emotional, and spiritual well-being. We practice being kind and compassionate to ourselves. A vital step in self-kindness is accepting ourselves just the way we are, including any thoughts and feelings about ourselves that are less than positive.

Do you ever catch yourself saying or thinking something negative about yourself? Maybe you've said something like, "I'm a loser," "I'm fat and out of shape," or "Wow, you are stupid!" Catching this negative self-talk and reframing it to a loving comment is an empowering self-acceptance and self-kindness practice. The next time you find yourself saying something unkind about yourself, pause and say to yourself, "I'm sorry. I love you just the way you are. I accept all of you. I will nourish you, cherish you, and not abuse you. I will honor the preciousness of this miracle life I've been given."

If negative self-talk is a big problem for you, try revisiting the exercise "Retrain Your Negative-Thinking Mind" from chapter 2. Negative self-talk is a version of negative thoughts. This exercise can help you reframe those thoughts and the negative feelings about yourself that come with them.

When we love ourselves, not only can we embody more love but we can also heal ourselves physically, mentally, and emotionally. Kelly McGonigal, psychologist and Stanford professor and researcher, says that when we have self-compassion we are happier, more optimistic, and have greater social connections.

There are many practices to help us build our ability to love ourselves. The affirmation exercise and the guided meditation at the end of this section are two good starting points. I'd also suggest trying Louise Hay's mirror practice. It may seem awkward at first to look yourself in the eyes and say, "I love you." But trust me: there is a deepening that happens the more you continue doing it.

If loving yourself seems really out of reach right now, try some of this chapter's other practices for embodying love first and then come back to this one.

Self-Love Affirmation

Put your hands on your heart area and take a deep breath. Feel into your heart area. Take another deep breath.

Say out loud the following affirmations:

You are loved.
You are cared for.
You are okay.

Breathe for a minute and then repeat these affirmations a few more times. Be present with what you are feeling.

Self-Love Guided Meditation

This meditation will help you cultivate self-love and compassion. Practice this meditation to feel healing love, warmth, and abundance in your life, knowing that the more you love yourself, the more love you have to give to others.

I invite you to close your eyes. Bring your attention to your breath.

Breathing in, notice how your body expands. Breathing out, notice your body recedes.

Become aware of any tension in your body and just breathe into that area for a moment.

Now feel the weight of your body being held by the ground, the floor, a chair, the bed—whatever you're sitting, standing, or lying on.

Let your body just soften and relax.

Feel your breath come into your body, and on your exhale, release again any tension you may be holding.

If your mind wanders, that is okay. Just come back to your breath.

Now visualize a golden light coming into your heart. This light is filling your entire heart area.

See this light getting bigger and brighter.

Feel your heart soften and expand.

You feel warmth and love in your heart.

Now visualize the sun. See rays of sunlight streaming into your heart. Feel this unconditional love energy.

This light now fills your chest and expands throughout your entire body.

Continue breathing in and breathing out.

This light is healing and bathing your body as it moves through you.

Whatever you need to let go of—physically, emotionally, spiritually—see it being released out of your body like gray smoke. See it leaving your body now.

Let go of any tension and stress. See the gray smoke drifting off.

Your body continues being bathed in this golden light that is within and all around you.

Surrender into this light and love.

Now say to yourself, either silently or out loud, "I love you. I really love you."

Feel this deep love in your heart and in your entire body. Take it in as you breathe in and out.

You are love.

Rest in this love for the next minute.

Bring your attention back to your breath, breathing in and out. When you are ready, you can gently open your eyes.

Feel an Embodied Connection with Something Greater

In my daily prayers, I offer thanks and gratitude for my life and say, "I love you, God—Father, Son, Holy Spirit—and archangels." When I say this and other prayers, I feel love as a soothing vibration in my heart, and a felt connection with God moves through me.

I believe our essence is love, and when we connect with something greater, no matter what we may call it, we're connecting with universal love. We're all extensions of this universal love. It is the highest vibrational energy, and when we consciously connect with it, we feel more love and aliveness.

Through this universal love, we can feel interconnected and one with all living beings and beings beyond. In my mystical experiences, I see spirits, including the spirits of the deceased, and I have felt the energy of love connecting me to them. I have also had brief encounters with angels in which the room has lit up, and a warmth and wonderment filled my being. These mystical experiences affirm for me that we are all expressions of this expansive love that is our true nature, and this love interconnects us all.

Like me, hundreds of people I companioned as a chaplain also experienced a felt sense of love in their connection with something greater. When people prayed, I saw and felt how they softened and how warmth entered their being. These feelings were even more palpable when someone was at the end of their life and taking their last breath. A warm glimmer and feeling of love often came over their face. I sensed, saw, and felt angelic guides present with people as their spirits departed from their body and flowed up and out of the room.

The second awakening practice invites each of us to connect with and experience something greater for ourselves. As you continue that practice, I invite you to tune in and specifically notice how your connection with something greater feels in your heart and body. Do you feel more warmth, more awe, more love in your being? Just be curious, open, and notice what is present in the moment as you explore.

"I Am Love" Prayer

The following prayer will help you feel into your relationship with something greater and open to universal love. If the words *Holy Spirit* do not resonate with you, fill in the language that speaks to your heart.

Thank you for this day.
Thank you for all the many ways you are present in my life.
Fill me with your love, light, and healing, Holy Spirit.
May your love flood through my body.
I am love. I am love. I am love.

Feel into Your Heart Center

Our heart area, or heart center, is located in the middle of our chest. It is often referred to as the heart chakra. *Chakra* is a Sanskrit word for an energy center in our bodies, and the Sanskrit name for the heart energy center is *Anahata*, which means "unstuck" or "unbeaten." This is the area where we feel empathy, love, forgiveness, and compassion. Here is where we feel connected to others. Here is where we may feel pain, brokenheartedness, unhappiness, and loneliness. It is in the heart center where we can feel all these feelings and let them move through us. When we do that, as discussed in chapter 2 and later in this chapter, our heart center opens and expands. When we cannot feel our feelings and allow them to move, our heart center closes. There is a flow of life and love in this energy center when our feelings are moving freely. There is a lack of flow and vitality in this center when we are stuck in our fear- or ego-based mind and feeling only grievances.

Just feeling into this flow of energy in your heart center takes you out of your mind. When you intentionally access the love flowing in your heart center, it can flow out through your body and beyond. Feeling this flowing movement of love in our being ignites a palpable aliveness, and our heart center expands to hold even more love.

You may have already started to feel this expansive feeling in your heart as you practiced coming back to the present moment and connecting with your soul in the first two awakening practices. There are also many additional ways to consciously and purposely feel into your heart center.

Kathy came in for a session with me because she wanted to feel more love. We discussed times in her life when she had felt love in her heart. She remembered how her grandmother had soothed and cared for her and had stroked her head at night. She described the love she felt with that memory as "a warm, opening sensation."

I then led Kathy in a guided heart-center meditation. At the end of it, she had a big smile and said, "I felt that." I encouraged her to practice the same meditation daily for a few weeks. When she walked into my office a month later, she shared, "I feel more love in my heart. I even now have tears at times when I'm watching TV. I feel more alive. Thank you."

Here is the meditation I shared with Kathy, plus two more exercises to help you feel into your heart center.

Come into Your Heart

This short meditation invites you to feel your heart center.

Start with coming into the present moment. Doing so allows you to step back from your mind.

Now breathe. Notice your breath coming in and out through your nostrils. You may want to close your eyes so you are not distracted.

Next, feel your clothes touching your skin. What does this sensation feel like?

When your mind starts to wander, just come back to your breath. Breathe in and breathe out.

Now breathe into your lower belly. Put your hand on it, and with your in-breath feel your hand rise. With your out-breath, feel your hand fall. You are stimulating your parasympathetic nervous system, and your body is automatically starting to relax.

As you continue this deep belly breathing, feel into your heart space. Let your heart speak. Let your heart open. Here is where the treasures of our soul and inner guidance arise.

What do you feel in your heart?

This question is not easy to answer when we are caught up in our mind and not able to tune in to our body. Maybe you have not connected with your body and heart for a long time. Yet our heart gives us so much information, if we take the time to listen.

Without any judgment, notice what arises. Maybe you feel a nudging, a stirring, or a pulling in a particular direction. Maybe you feel a sense of calmness. Can you name what is arising?

Whatever arises, open to it. Let the feeling have space. Feel it. Breathe into it. Feelings are not permanent, and when you feel them, they move through you. As you let them move through you, you create space for love, joy, peace, and guidance to come in, one breath at a time.

Continue being with whatever arises for the next few minutes.

When you are ready, bring your attention back to your body. Feel your body being supported by a chair or the floor. Then you can gently open your eyes.

Mantra and Toning for Your Heart Center

This exercise will help you feel your heart center.

Start by toning the word *yum*, a Sanskrit syllable and sound associated with heart center. Feel the vibrational energy of this sound in your heart center. Toning the word *yum* can bring this area into balance.

Now put your hands over your heart area. Feel the warmth of your hands and breathe. Our bodies always respond to physical touch. Let your body soften and relax.

Say silently or out loud, "I am love." This is the mantra of our heart center.

Notice and feel love in your heart area. Feel this love expand and fill your entire chest. Then feel it move through your entire body.

Drop your hands. Bring your focus back to your breath, breathing in and breathing out.

On your out-breath, tone the sound *yum* again, or sound the word *ah*, another sound of the heart center.

Practice sounding *yum* or *ah* for the next couple of minutes. Notice the vibration in your chest area and in your entire body. You are awakening your heart center, the seat of your soul.

When you are ready, stop toning. Just notice what is present in your body right now.

End by the saying the phrase "I am" out loud or silently.

Journey to Your Heart Guided Meditation

The following guided meditation, based on one shared by Liz Simpson in her 2013 book *The Book of Chakra Healing*, invites you to see and heal your heart. I once practiced this meditation every day for a month because I was determined to feel my heart more. After a month, I noticed a fluttering in my heart and felt a deepening in my being. Try it yourself and see what you think.

Allow your mind and body to relax. Feel peace come through your body. If thoughts come into your mind, let them pass and come back to your breath, breathing in and breathing out.

You are about to take a journey to your heart. As you do, acknowledge the feelings that may arise, but don't dwell on them. Know that you are safe, protected, and loved.

Imagine yourself standing in a beautiful meadow, surrounded by wildflowers. You can hear birds a little way off. You can feel the warmth of the sun on your face and body. You know you are completely safe.

From the edge of the meadow, you walk into a forest. Soon you see a clearing ahead. As you walk into the clearing, you see a large area of bare ground, with scattered fallen green leaves around it. As you walk closer, you see your heart lying there on the ground.

Pay attention to what you see. How does your heart look? Is it beating? Is it shrunken or bleeding because you give too much to others? Is it cold or covered in ice because you are closed off? Is it discolored or lifeless because you feel withdrawn and closed off? Does it have an irregular heartbeat because you feel a lot of anxiety? Just notice what you see without any judgment.

Give your heart whatever it needs. If it is bleeding, put your hands on it to stop blood flow. If it looks discolored, lifeless, or shrunken, send it love.

If it is cold, surround it with warm heaters. If it is encased in ice, chip away the ice. If it is beating irregularly, gently hold your hand on it to calm it.

Spend the next minutes giving your heart what it needs.

When you have finished, send healing love into your heart.

Know that you can return to this clearing and heal your heart whenever you want to.

Take a few deep breaths. Feel the weight of your body supported by whatever surface you are sitting, standing, or lying on. When you are ready, you can open your eyes.

Hold Gratitude

Gratitude elicits a strong, palpable vibration in our body. Feeling gratitude in our body—maybe in our gut or our chest area—for even a few minutes strengthens our immune system and uplifts our body, mind, and spirit. As we hold gratitude in our heart, our heart softens, and we grow our capacity to feel more love.

I've found that a daily gratitude practice is a powerful way to feel more love and thankfulness in my body. When I do it in the morning, the high-vibrational energy begins coursing through my body and sets the tone for my whole day. It also sets me up to notice and feel more gratitude during even seemingly mundane moments. My heart always softens with gratitude, for example, when I get into bed and see my dogs. I push Gigi over a little so there is room for me to lay my head on my pillow. Then I look over to see Bella smashed up against my sleeping husband, snoring. Bella's under the covers, with only her head popping out from the warm, soft down comforter. The sight is heartwarming and a bit funny. The quiet is present, the snoring is present, and I feel warmth and calmness. I feel grateful. In this moment, all is okay. The upheaval and unrest of the world drop away. Prayers of thankfulness come flooding through me.

What moments in your day stir up a feeling of thankfulness in your being?

Whether you find moments of gratitude in the flow of daily living or you create them through a gratitude practice, may you savor and embody them in your heart.

Morning Gratitude Practice

Take a few minutes at the beginning of your day, before you even get out of bed, to hold gratitude in your heart.

Bring to mind all the things you are grateful for in your life. Feel the thankfulness in your heart and in your body. Savor this feeling in your body for a few minutes.

If you like, you can also hold your arms and hands in a prayer position in front of your heart area. Say, "Thank you," as you breathe in and breathe out. Feel the weight of your body being held by whatever surface you're lying, sitting, or standing on. Feel your breath come in and out of your body.

Gratitude Meditation

This short meditation builds a feeling of gratitude in your body. I've found it to be a wonderful way to start the day, but you can practice it at any time.

Allow your body to soften. Just let yourself be.

Allow your awareness to move to your breath. Become aware of your in-breath and your out-breath. Notice how your body expands on the in-breath and recedes on the out-breath.

Open to these statements of gratitude as you say them out loud or silently:

> *I am grateful to be alive.*
> *I am grateful for my body, my breath, my health.*
> *I am grateful for my family and friends.*
> *I am grateful for my food and the home that I live in.*
> *I am grateful for this new day—for the chance to start anew, with an open mind and heart and spirit.*

Continue breathing in and breathing out.

Now say out loud or silently:

> *I am grateful for all I have learned up to this moment, including the challenges in my life that have opened my heart.*
> *I am grateful for all the support I receive from the seen and unseen worlds. I am not alone.*
> *I am grateful for nature—for the trees, bushes, flowers, mountains, rivers, lakes, and oceans that soothe my soul.*
> *I am grateful for love, laughter, and the many small wonders in my daily life.*
> *I am grateful for all the living creatures, big and small, in this world. I am grateful for all the immense beauty that is ever present.*

Now you can name, silently or out loud, whatever else may come to mind that you are grateful for.

Continue breathing in and breathing out. When you are ready, say:

> I breathe in love, feeling it come through my body, and breathe out any
> unrest.
> I feel warmth and gratitude in my heart.
> I am grateful for life.

Continue focusing on your breath, breathing in and breathing out, until you're ready to close.

Remember Times of Deep Love

We can use our memories of times we felt deep love for someone, or felt their deep love for us, to expand our ability to embody love. Bringing to mind those times is a way of reminding ourselves that we have indeed experienced giving or receiving love, and it will call up a felt sense of love in our body and being again. This practice is especially useful when we feel a void or a lack of love.

Love comes in many forms, and if we are lucky, we get a few great teachers during our lives. My dogs have been some of my biggest spiritual teachers. One of the most important lessons they've taught me is how to receive unconditional love. Specific memories of my past and current dogs are ones I turn to when I want to feel a visceral sense of love.

Lulu, my beloved bichon, had been by my side ever since she joined our household at five months old. She slept snuggled in bed with me every night and deferred to me for all her needs. My family joked that she only wanted to be with me. Throughout her life, whenever we had gazed into each other's eyes, I'd felt pure love, warmth, and contentment, and my heart had expanded. Few things were as delightful as coming home from a difficult day as a hospice chaplain to be greeted by the light of this precious creature. She had made my life complete.

In August 2018, thirteen-year-old Lulu developed an infection, and her lungs filled up with fluid. We took her to the veterinary ICU, but the vet said there was nothing they could do. Holding her in my arms, I felt like my heart was being ripped out of my chest. Just moments before the vet was to give her a sedative to help her pass, she awakened, turned her head, and stared straight into my eyes. I gasped and looked away. Fear coursed through my body as I saw the great life force in her eyes and realized it was about to leave. I prayed over her as she buried her head in my stomach. The injection was administered, and she peacefully left her little, white, furry body.

As I sobbed, I felt my heart expand and overflow with the limitless love I felt for Lulu. My bond with her, I realized, was one of those once-in-a-lifetime experiences.

To this day, whenever I think of her, my heart warms and expands. She continues to teach me about love now from the other side. I feel a deeper sense of love and its luminous power in my heart whenever I remember and savor the love I felt, and still feel, for her.

Remembering Love

Think back to a time when you felt deep love for someone or received love from someone. It could be a family member, a pet—any loved one. It doesn't matter who it was; what matters is that the love you gave or received was so moving that you felt it in your whole being.

Take a few minutes and remember this time. Feel it in your heart. Savor it. Let the feeling expand in your heart center and move through your body.

Spend a few minutes feeling this love in your body.

Share Love with Challenging People

As my friend Laurie noted, when she shares love with others, she feels even more love and warmth and aliveness move through her. It is typically not that difficult to share love with our loved ones. It is also relatively easy to extend love and kindness to people who are kind and friendly to us. But how can we practice sharing love with others when they are not kind to us or have treated us poorly?

It is possible. I know from firsthand experience that sharing love with challenging people can be a potent way to expand the love we feel in our own body and being, regardless of how they may treat us.

In one of my jobs, I had a few challenging colleagues. I'd walk into the conference room, and they seemed to pretend I didn't exist. They'd lower their voices and continue talking about our mutual patients without any regard for me or my own work with that patient. Then they'd talk about weekend social plans while barely acknowledging that I had said hello.

I agonized over how I was going to work with them. I decided not to change my outward behavior, but every time I was in meetings with them, I'd visualize love and light flowing into their bodies. The more I chose to hold love and embody love in my heart, the more I was able to continue sending love and light to these colleagues in my mind. As a result, my heart opened more, and I was able to feel more love. And interestingly, over time, these colleagues softened and became more friendly and inclusive.

> *Love is a state of being. You begin to love people because they just are. . . . When you live in love, you see love everywhere you look. You are literally in love with everyone you look at.*
> —Ram Dass, Cookbook for Awakening

Visualizing love surrounding someone also helped me extend love to my father-in-law, Jim, in his dying moments.

Jim had never learned unconditional love as a child. His father had died in World War II, when Jim was two years old. His mother was an alcoholic who was not present in his life. Jim had spent his entire life seeking love, external recognition, and support. His life looked glamorous from the outside, with money, a successful business, and a family. But inside him there was a lack of love stemming from his early childhood needs that were never addressed. As an adult, he was a narcissist and an alcoholic. Over the twenty-four years that I had been in his family, he had often unintentionally pushed us away. We never knew what mood he would be in at family gatherings, and if he didn't like how a particular conversation was going or what was said, he'd get angry and at times outright mean. He wanted things to go his way, and when they didn't, he'd get agitated and upset.

Yet he deserved and needed to be loved deeply. Love was all that mattered as he lay dying in his cold, austere ICU room.

My children, Scott, and I had gathered around his bed. The breathing tube in his throat was removed, and he opened his eyes briefly and made a little eye contact with us. We all told him, "I love you." I thanked him for all he had done for our family. He had tears in his eyes.

I visualized white light and love moving through his body. I prayed for God's healing spirit to comfort Jim as he was letting go. His other son, Jimmy, arrived, and we all sat vigil around Jim. We shared many family stories around his hospital bed.

He died six hours later, peacefully, with family gathered around him.

I believe Jim felt love all around him in his final hours, and this helped him peacefully let go. The palpable feeling of love in the room also gave us, his family, a deeper sense of the meaning and power of love. I felt more love move through my heart and whole being by sharing love with him, one of the most challenging people in my life, that day.

Extending Love Exercise

Here's an exercise you can do the next time you encounter someone who is dismissive, rude, off-putting, unpleasant, or unfriendly to you.

First, quickly tune in to what you are thinking and feeling. Can you name the thought that is arising? Can you name the feeling that is arising?

Now take a deep breath. Feel into this feeling. Where are you feeling it in your body? Be open. Be curious.

Next instead of changing your behavior or being critical or rude back to this person, decide to do the opposite: Share kindness. Smile at them. Ask how their day is going.

Notice how extending this kind energy feels for you in the moment. Then after you've left the situation, notice how you feel.

These steps may seem like a lot to do if the encounter is short, such as when you are standing in a checkout line with people behind you. You might instead just notice the unrest arising in your body and choose to take a deep breath. Then you can respond to this challenging person with kindness and see what happens.

If the person is not open to kindness or doesn't respond in kind, don't take it personally. Instead, you can use my friend Laurie's approach: bless the person in your mind and move on.

Let Go of the Judgment Habit

Judging others keeps us from fully embodying love. The more judgment we hold, the less space there is for love and universal life energy to come through us. When we judge others, we become more deeply entrenched in our ego mind.

Our ego mind loves to compare, contrast, and critique others, especially when it feels threatened or less than. Judging others makes it feel better. This good feeling is usually fleeting and temporary, and when it passes, we are left with feeling a quagmire of negative thoughts and difficult feelings. Our being becomes engulfed in their energy, and it doesn't feel good. Feeling poorly again, our mind turns again to judgment to feel better, reinforcing the harmful cycle.

The first step of getting out of the judgment habit is to catch yourself when you want to critique or judge someone. Take a deep breath. Instead of getting lost in what you're thinking or feeling about the other person, take a mental step back. Ask what is arising within yourself. What is getting triggered? How do you feel threatened? Breathe into the thoughts and feelings, as well as the negative energy that comes with them. Looking inward; reflecting on the angst, unrest, or other difficult feelings you find; and letting them move through you is how you will feel better—not by judging others.

Afterward, see if you can feel into the love you already have in your heart. Tapping into it and letting it move through your body will help you release any more of the negative thoughts, difficult feelings, and negative energy, and opens your heart even more to love.

Our ego mind can also flare up when we find ourselves on the receiving end of another's judgment. Our ego mind gets hooked, and we are ready to jump in and react to the person. By choosing to step back and not engage with our ego mind, we give ourselves room to look within and focus on feeling our own feelings rather than getting lost in our reaction to the other person's judgment.

We can't control what other people think of us. We can only control how we respond.

Other people's judgment cannot change our essence. What other people think of us and how they treat us are not about us, but about them. Their judgmental words and actions are a direct reflection of their inner world. Their judgment means their inner mirror is cloudy. When someone holds judgment about us, they hold this judgment inside themselves. They hold unrest and pain in their heart, compromising their ability to embody love.

I have learned that taking in the energy of other people's judgment closes our heart. The more we practice embodying love, the more we can hold our own power. Then, when the arrows of other people's judgment come toward us, they just fly by. We can remain open-hearted and feel more deeply alive, no matter what others think, say, or do. It is empowering and freeing when we realize that other people's negative judgments about us don't have to affect us.

As I was writing this book, an old friend had been critiquing me, my life, and my business—basically, how I was showing up in the world. Her judgment felt unsettling. My ego mind felt hurt. Even though I knew her judgment was a reflection of her inner world, my mind spent a lot of time wondering why she was judging me.

Eventually, I realized trying to figure it out was only hurting me. Nothing good was coming of it. I stopped looking at the situation with my ego mind and dropped into my heart center. From my heart's viewpoint, I felt gratitude for my friend. She had given me a lot and enabled me to become the person I am today, living my deep inner truth. At the same time, I realized our friendship had changed and was no longer working well. I listened deeply within, felt the angst and sadness I found there, and breathed into these feelings and released them. More space opened within me, and I felt more freedom. Instead of contracting, my heart expanded, and I felt universal love flow through me.

Release Buried Emotions

I tossed and turned throughout the night. My mind kept reviewing the book chapters I'd finally finished and submitted to my editor after months of hard work. I dreamed all night of those chapters and the story of my childhood illness included in them.

Upon awakening in the morning, I felt anger. How strange to wake up angry! This was a new experience for me.

I lay in bed and touched into the feeling. I felt the anger bubbling up. What was I angry about?

As I breathed into it, an image surfaced. I saw myself as a child, alone in the hospital, and no one was telling me what was happening to me. In the forty-plus years since that experience, I'd never felt anger about it before. My mind wanted to analyze this anger, but I decided to just feel it.

I continued breathing in and out, letting the anger come up. Then, underneath it, I found fear. A thread of terror ran through my body as if I were eleven years old again. Tears swelled in my eyes. I felt the same fear I'd felt then: *am I going to live?*

When we don't feel our feelings in the moment they arise, they can get stuck in our body, mind, and spirit. Pushing them down or suppressing them again and again only creates layers of buried emotions within us. Those buried emotions might seem to be dormant—that is, until something triggers them. Then we can see just how much this vast array of unfelt emotions are affecting us, even though we may not know it. The energy of these buried, stuck emotions takes up space in the container of our being, reducing the amount of room we have for love.

Though I'd had a profound awakening during my years of hospital treatments, there were still some feelings from the experience that I hadn't felt, released, and integrated. I had been able to open into and release some of these buried feeling in therapy as an adult, and I had done a lot more deep inner work over the years. Yet here was another layer coming to the surface.

Emotions are not permanent—not even ones that we have suppressed for years. Releasing buried emotions often happens little by little, layer by layer, over time. If we let ourselves feel each new layer as it surfaces, it will dissipate and move through us. As I lay in bed, I understood that I needed to release this pent-up anger and fear that I still had within me. I continued breathing in and out as I felt again all that fear, along with the stark loneliness, the emptiness, that had come with being so young and fragile and alone.

Then, just as it did when I was eleven, a warmth entered. I felt a peace that was not of this world. My body softened. I remembered how a presence had come into me as a child and how it comforted me. Now again, more than forty-five years later, I was feeling this presence. I knew again I wasn't alone.

My tears turned into tears of gratitude. Prayers of thankfulness came through me. Like I had as a child, I felt grateful to be alive.

Coming back to the present moment and becoming a witness to our thoughts and feelings, as described in the exercise "Retrain Your Negative-Thinking Mind" in chapter 2, can help us feel and release each layer of anger, fear, or other long-buried feelings. If the buried feelings are too much for you to feel on your own, please seek professional help. Each time you feel and release another layer of buried emotions, more space opens in your body and being to feel more love.

Embrace Forgiveness

When I was eight years old, my father stood inches from my face and yelled, "You are nothing!" My spirit was crushed.

I remember this comment and others like them being thrown at me throughout my childhood. All I could do at the time was bury the deep pain, hurt, fear, anger, and confusion I felt.

Going to therapy in my late twenties helped me process the layers of these buried feelings. Again and again, I opened into the pain, anger, bitterness, and other difficult emotions; unearthed another layer; and released it. Finally, I reached a point where I simply did not want to feel any of these feelings in my body at all. I just didn't want to carry them with me anymore. A deep knowing surfaced from within: if I wanted to feel more space in my being and embody more love, I needed to forgive my father for his verbal abuse.

Forgiveness does not mean forgetting what happened. Forgiveness is not for the person who hurt us. Forgiveness is for self-healing. I knew that hanging on to pain, anger, bitterness, and other difficult emotions in our body, mind, and spirit only hurts us. So every time another layer of these feelings came to the surface, not only did I feel through it and release it but I also prayed to feel forgiveness for my father.

As I did, my heart opened more, and I began to feel free. I came to truly forgive him. As a result, I felt more peace and love in my heart.

Over time, I began to see that his verbal abuse, though it had harmed me, was never about me. I saw how he had done the best he could. Forgiveness opened a door that allowed me to see him as a complex man capable of both great fear and great love. With his verbal abuse, he had projected his fear onto the people he loved. Yet when I was eleven, he had also worn a toupee in solidarity with me the first day I went to school wearing a wig, after I'd lost my hair to chemotherapy. "I thought we could go through this together," he'd said as he drove me to school. I'd felt his deep love and companionship, and it helped me through a difficult time in my life.

I was with my father as he took his last breaths. My heart felt wide open and free, and the deep love between us flowed through the bedroom. I said goodbye and "I love you" while his spirit left his body.

I thought I had released the pain of my father's verbal abuse, so I was taken aback when, just recently, an experience with a few family members retriggered it. *Ah, there is more work to do here*, I said to myself.

I developed laryngitis. Not being able to talk for days, I was able to be very quiet and look within. Every time a thread of pain resurfaced, I breathed into the present moment. I breathed into the tightness I felt in my chest and found its source. I breathed into the felt pain. I felt again the anger of being silenced. As I breathed into it, it moved. I felt an opening, a release in my body. I then visualized sunlight flooding my heart and moving through my entire body. As I breathed out, I visualized the angst and unrest floating out of my body as gray smoke.

After several fifteen-minute sessions of this exercise, I felt peace in my entire body. My breath felt longer and deeper.

I then practiced forgiveness, saying, "I love you. I bless you. I release you," to all family involved in my life, past and present.

A softness entered—a letting go. I felt love and compassion for myself, my father, and all the family members involved in the recent conflict.

Complex relationships, such as those we often have with our family, are opportunities for us to practice forgiveness and thus grow and learn to embody more love. It can be very challenging to forgive our family members when they have hurt us. But at the end of the day, if we don't forgive and relinquish the pain we are holding, the pain continues to hurt us. Forgiveness frees us from that pain and helps us embody more love.

I invite you to look inward and see if there is any buried pain, anger, bitterness, or other difficult feelings that are holding you back from embodying love. Maybe you're not ready to forgive the people whose actions contributed to those feelings, but is there an opening? Can you offer a prayer or intention to your inner wisdom or to universal energy—"Help me to forgive"? Start there. Just this step opens the door to forgiveness. Asking for help starts you down the path of forgiveness.

Sometimes the person we need to forgive is ourselves. Maybe we need to forgive ourselves for behavior we later regret, something we said that we wished we hadn't, or treating someone with little kindness.

To begin forgiving yourself, bring the situation into your consciousness, choose to let go of any harsh inner self-critique, release any internal anguish or other difficult feelings, and offer a blessing to any people involved in the situation. Remind yourself that no one is perfect, things happen, and offering yourself forgiveness is a way of embodying more love.

> *It's one of the greatest gifts you can give*
> *yourself, to forgive. Forgive everybody.*
> —Maya Angelou

When we forgive, we are choosing to prioritize love over fear, anger, pain, bitterness, and judgment. When we forgive another or ourselves, we heal and empower ourselves, and we are able to embody more love.

Forgiveness Exercise

If you have a hard time forgiving someone, try this exercise.

Look in the mirror and say out loud, "I forgive you, (name of the person)."

Just be open to what surfaces. You will quickly start to see what's holding you back from forgiving that person.

Send loving-kindness energy to the person you want to forgive by saying, "May you be at peace," or a similar phrase. You may even send them a blessing.

Finally, breathe into your body. Whatever feelings arise, let them have space to be as you continue to breathe. Your body knows the truth, and only when you let the feelings arise and move through you can you release them and heal.

Fully Embodying Love

Irene, a small, elderly woman, was sitting on the couch as I walked through the front door of her home. She had a prayer shawl covering her frail shoulders and thin arms, and she gave me a big, warm smile. She had an uncanny glow about her, I noticed, as I sat down in the chair next to her.

"I have had a good life. I have no regrets. I know God is with me. I am okay," Irene said. She reached out her hand to hold mine.

"I pray several times a day," she continued. She pulled over her prayer box that was sitting on the couch next to her and showed me her large stack of prayers.

My eyes widened. I was mesmerized by this big box and what looked like a large pile of well-worn collected prayers. I was just as fascinated by the warm, golden glow that extended from Irene and filled the room.

"I have told God that I am ready. I have learned that all you need in life is love. I love everyone. I love my family and friends. Love is the answer," Irene shared.

We spent the entire visit talking about love, her family, and her friends. She had her share of hardships in life, and the power sustaining her was her love for God and love for her family. "Opening and feeling the love that is all around is what life is all about," she said.

On the next few visits, we read a wide range of the favorite prayers she had collected over the past forty years. Irene continued to talk about her understanding that love is the answer to all questions.

"I have no fear of death. I know God is with me. All you take with you is the love in your heart and your ability to love. This is what it means to be alive," she kept saying.

Two weeks after my first visit, I received a page from the hospice staff, who said Irene was actively dying and near the end of her life. I arrived and was led to her bedroom. She turned her head slightly in my direction and wiggled her hand. I sat on the side of her bed and held her hand. A slight smile came across her face; her love was palpable. The sun was shining through the window, and light fell on the side of her face. She looked radiant and beautiful. Just being in her presence, I felt my heart expand and love flow through my body.

"All is well. You are ready. God is here," I told her. I read one of her favorite prayers and looked deeply into her brown eyes. I smiled and thanked her for being a teacher for me.

A tear fell down the side of her cheek. She squeezed my hand, and she closed her eyes.

Upon leaving her house, I knew she did not have long to live. Death felt very close, and she was ready to go. I thought to myself, *So this is what it feels like to have a wide-open heart—to feel love so completely that all else drops away, including any fear.*

She passed late that evening.

Facing straight into death with no fear but with love and an open heart, Irene exemplified what embodying love looks like. She had learned to fully accept the moment and let go of any fear or unrest. She had mastered the biggest life lesson: life is about fully embodying love.

Thinking and talking about love only takes us so far. If we can't *feel* love, we can't feel fully alive. When we embody love, like Irene did, we can experience and feel the fullness of being alive right now. When we live from our heart, we experience the deep love that we are. We touch into and find our soul, where the Divine, the universe, resides and moves through us.

Embodying love will help you choose more love and give more love, and this love reinforces itself.

We are called to love, and what we take with us at death is our capacity to love.

You don't have to wait until the end of your life to feel more love. You can learn to embody more love in your being right now. Embodying love will awaken you to the preciousness of being alive.

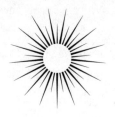

6

THE FIFTH PRACTICE

Hold Openness

OPENNESS IS OUR NATURAL STATE. Openness is the opposite of resistance. When we experience life with openness, we feel alive. Our essence and power flow freely through us.

If you've started working with the first four awakening practices, you may already be feeling more open and alive. Being in the present moment instead of lost in our mind creates a felt sense of spaciousness within. Connecting with something greater opens us to our soul and an expansive feeling of oneness. When we trust, we fully accept this moment, and we open ourselves to the flow and possibilities of life. When we embody love, our essence naturally opens. This fifth practice encourages us to continue to hold that sense of openness as we move through life's challenges.

During difficult times, it is easy to stay in our ego mind, which will usually try to fix and control the situation. If it can't, it can shut us down, keeping us from being in our body and experiencing the flow of life and our emotions in the moment. Although our nervous system's freeze response may cause us to close down to help us survive a crisis, this response is designed to be temporary and short-lived. Living full time in this state is not healthy. In our efforts to avoid the challenges of life, we may create a protective shell around us, like a crab, and live inside this shell. We harden ourselves. This is the opposite of holding openness.

When we hold openness, there is the potential to survive extremely difficult experiences without shutting down. That in itself is growth. In other circumstances, holding openness allows a difficult experience to be a potential awakening opportunity.

Holding openness is an invitation to experience whatever is happening in the moment with a little space and curiosity. It is a conscious choice: We decide we are going to stay present and feel what is arising in the moment, experience the energy of it, and not close ourselves off to it. We decide to keep the door open and live into the unknown, even if it is hard.

If we are able to allow even a small opening, a softening enters. From there, we can continue to feel into our heart and soul, our essence, and the preciousness of life.

The invitation of openness is to fall into the infinity of your true nature. It is from here that true freedom can begin.
—Amoda Maa, Falling Open in a World Falling Apart

A friend once said to me, "I want to keep learning and growing, but I don't want to go through anything hard." In so many words, she was telling the universe, "I want to learn and grow but on my terms." Instead of holding openness, she was trying to control how her life would unfold. In doing so, she closed herself off from life.

The idea that we hold openness when we are in the thick of a very difficult experience can be very hard to comprehend and accept. Some of us, like my friend, may say, "Enough," and try to dictate to the universe our growth terms. Others of us may swallow our feelings and close up, in trying to avoid our hardships.

Our challenging experiences of life can help us awaken, if we let them. It takes courage and strength, but when we're able to hold openness during the hard times, our heart and soul open even more, opening us even further to the fullness of life. Walking through fire, we soften, we may be seared, and then we melt. We come out on the other side, grossly and vibrantly alive. This is the path of awakening.

Going with the Flow and Finding Balance

Holding openness allows us to find balance and move with the flow of whatever is happening in our lives—positive or negative, challenging or mundane, everyday or extraordinary.

When we open into the energy and movement of what is present, we allow universal life force energy to flow through us. We move and flow with the energy of life, instead of limiting, resisting, or trying to stop it, or hiding away in a shell, disengaged from it.

Holding openness amid the joys and sorrows in life is a balancing act. Balance exists when we're open, present, and not going to extremes as life is happening within and around us. We consciously choose to take in what is life giving and let go of what is not.

I relearned the value of holding openness after my husband came home from the hospital ICU with a pacemaker and a diagnosis of a rare heart condition. Uncertainty was front and center in our lives, and this uncertainty, coupled with my intense hospice job, which was a continual contemplation of life and death, created what felt like a tipping point. The question kept coming through me: "How am I going to go back to carrying a pager and working with dying patients when I'm living in such uncertainty with my husband?"

I found balance in being open to my inner experience, being curious about it, and letting my feelings move through me. I kept leaning into the flow of life rather than resisting it. Practicing connecting with God, deep listening, and embodying love, along with my meditation practice and the support of my family and close friends, helped me stay open and balanced amid the palpable uncertainty we were living with.

You can't stop the waves, but you can learn to surf.
—Jon Kabat-Zinn, Wherever You Go, There You Are

Holding openness allows us to keep our balance as we ride the waves of life's ups and downs. Staying present in this moment and living in our heart and soul, instead of our mind, also help us keep our balance when it feels like we're teetering on choppy waters. In moments of stagnation, coming back into our body and practicing acceptance and trust will help us allow life to begin to flow through us again. Instead of pushing, resisting, or controlling each moment, we are opening and allowing. Opening to those things that give us support allows us to stay in the flow of life and continue to awaken.

When we hold openness, we are able to allow life to move through us. When life moves through us, we are less likely to close down. Our mind is less likely to hold on to fear and to try to control everything. We realize that control is really an illusion.

Those who flow as life flows know they need no other force.
—*Lao Tzu,* The Way of Life According to
Lao Tzu *(translated by Witter Bynner)*

When we let go of our resistance to the flow of life, endless possibilities arise. Life is suddenly not defined by our limited ego mind. We open into wonder.

My mother-in-law, Karen, reinforced for me how holding openness can help us balance and move with the flow of life even in the face of death. During the year she was navigating inoperable pancreatic cancer, I accompanied her on all her appointments with doctors and many alternative healers. During a visit with our shamanic practitioner, Michael, he asked her, "Are you going with the river or trying to go upstream?"

Karen said, "I am going with the river."

Her words touched my soul. Instead of resisting, she had chosen to hold openness. She had chosen to accept what was happening to her and flow with it, moment by moment.

Because Karen was able to hold openness, a whole new life emerged for her. Her previous love of shopping and material things dropped away; her sense of aliveness grew stronger. Each day, she opened into the preciousness of the moment, surfed each wave, and became more vibrantly alive.

When we can keep the door cracked open, we are able to go with the flow of life. We stop fighting the currents, both inner and outer. We stop pushing and start allowing. We begin to understand that there is more to this big life than meets the eye.

If you let go a little, you will have a little peace. If you
let go a lot, you will have a lot of peace. If you let go
completely, you will know complete peace and freedom.
—Ajahn Chah, A Still Forest Pool

Once you start moving with the flow of life on a regular basis instead of fighting it, you will find it is easier to stay balanced and hold openness. You will feel freedom, spaciousness, and vibrant aliveness.

Let Go, Let Be

Try the following guided meditation when you are feeling stagnant and closed. Practice it and see if you feel an opening, a little more space to feel life and go with life's flow.

Become aware of any tension in your body and just breathe into that area for a moment, breathing in and breathing out.

Allow your mind and body to relax. If thoughts come into your mind, let them pass and come back to your breath—your in-breath, your out-breath.

Breathe into your heart. Feel it open, soften, expand.

Breathe into your belly. Feel it rise on the in-breath and fall on the out-breath.

Let your body relax. Let go of any tension, any unease.

Now visualize a river flowing into an ocean. The water of the river is calm, expansive, a clear blue, a soothing temperature. There is a flow to it.

Know that you are the water, flowing smoothly.

You are flowing around the rocks that lead to the ocean, touching the river banks, pooling for a moment in a small crevice and then flowing beyond.

Let go, let be.

Go with the flow. *Be* the flow.

There is slow movement, a fluidity.

You feel a sense of spaciousness, ease, peace—a sense of aliveness.

You flow up to a large branch. You move up and around it and over it.

You move into a stillness, a spaciousness, a sense of just being.

Let go of any unrest. Just notice what is present.

Trust this spaciousness you are feeling.

Surrender to it.

Surrender into this moment.

You may experience a ripple, a gentle wave.

Ride the wave. Let it carry you.

Let go, let be.

You move back into stillness.

In this moment, you are okay.

Feel peace and ease within and around you.

Feel a sense of floating, a calmness, a letting go.

Rest in this peace.

Rest in this stillness.

Ask Something Greater for Help

If you're having trouble holding openness, ask for help. God, universal life energy, whatever we may call the something greater we are all connected to—it is ever present, and when we open to it and allow it to flow through us, we can hold more openness during challenging times.

Reaching out to God and angels, such as the archangel Michael, helped Karen hold openness as she faced her cancer diagnosis and impending death. She chose to have faith, and she felt supported by it. I could not feel any fear in her as I walked with her through her many appointments with doctors and other health practitioners.

Active faith gives us deep roots in this something greater. With these deep roots, we become like a strong tree, able to sway with the winds yet not break. With these roots, we can weather the storms of our lives.

Like Karen, my ninety-four-year-old mother has a connection with something greater that helps her during challenging times. Her daily prayer practice and strong faith in God has enabled her to stay open in the face of aging and physical limitations, as well as the coronavirus pandemic.

When the pandemic began, she stopped going out in public, except for a few doctor appointments and to get her hair done once a week in an empty salon, where her hairdresser wore a mask. Yet she remained cheerful and full of life. When I'd visit her, she would recount the range of friends and neighbors she has recently talked with on the phone.

Out of curiosity, I'd ask, "In a given week, do you ever find yourself worrying?"

"No," she'd reply.

"Do you find yourself having moments of feeling anxiety?"

"No." She'd shrug. "I really don't. I have adapted."

I'd look at her neatly coiffed hair, her stylish blue cat-eye eyeglasses, and the smile on her face, and I'd marvel. I could feel her strength, fortitude, and unwavering faith. I'd feel a nudging inside me that said, "Take note of her deep faith and felt guidance." I am grateful to see this teaching right in front of my eyes.

Prayer for Help

The following is a short, simple prayer requesting help with holding openness. Practice saying it on a regular basis, but let go of any desired outcome. Just take note of what happens. You just may be surprised by what you experience.

Help me to stay open.
Help me to hear your guidance.
Pour your spirit through me.
May I feel your presence.

Feeling into Fear

When we are in fear, it is easy to shut down. It can be hard to hold openness during challenging times because our fear makes us want to do the opposite.

Fear comes to us as thoughts in our mind and sensations in our body. It is a primal, visceral feeling that often stems from feeling threatened physically, emotionally, or spiritually. Fear is a natural emotion and serves a good purpose: to help us mobilize when we are in danger. The problem is, we can feel fearful when there is no actual danger. In these cases, instead of keeping us safe, our fearful thoughts and feelings can knock us off-balance and even immobilize us. If our fear becomes a long-standing habit, our nervous system stays dysregulated, and we begin to live in a fight-or-flight or freeze response. This chronic fear can lead to depression and anxiety and create imbalances in our health and well-being that lead to disease.

When we get stuck thinking of the past or the future, fear can grab hold of our ego mind. Our minds are so powerful, and fear and negative thinking can easily take over our mind. It is easy to swing back and forth between a fearful thought to a fearful feeling and thus get stuck in a limbic loop, as discussed in chapter 2. If we don't interrupt that limbic loop, it only becomes stronger. When we are feeling too much fear too often, we might close our hearts and shut down to try to avoid it. Our unfelt fear becomes buried within us, only to be triggered later. Buried fear may come out as judgment, blaming, anger, and reactivity.

Many of us fear death, the unknown, or uncertainty. We often have at least one big fear from our early childhood that is easily triggered again and again. Maybe you notice you have an ongoing fear of something, someone, a situation, and your fearful perception turns into a chronic fearful thought or feeling. You get stuck in that fear the way a leaf might get on a rock as it's floating on a river; the water of life continues moving, but you can't flow with it.

We can't think our fear away. It is through feeling fear when it arises that we move through it.

My ability to hold openness in the midst of great fear was suddenly put to the test one day in early May 2020. Scott, who'd had a cough for over a month, awakened with a 103-degree fever. He was already at a high risk for catching the coronavirus because of his heart condition and the immunosuppressant drugs he takes for it. I drove him to the doors of the ER, hugged him, and said goodbye. Fear surrounded me as I watched him walk into the hospital alone.

While waiting at home to hear the results from Scott's first Covid test, I called my daughter, Adria, in Miami. As we were talking, I heard gunshots on her end of the phone.

Adria hung up, ran to her apartment balcony, hid in a corner, and called the police. Then she called me back, sobbing. My heart started racing. I tried to be present with her. We breathed together over the phone, and I said silent prayers. Within minutes, Adria could hear police sirens nearby, and then police officers entered her high-rise apartment building.

I hung up the phone. All the fear I'd been holding at bay poured through me, and I broke down crying. The fear was intense, but I surrendered to it. I knew I had to let it out.

Ten minutes later, Adria called back and said the police were on her floor. The shooter had been right outside her door, firing at the door of another apartment.

Minutes later, I got a call from Scott. "My first Covid test is negative," he said.

Sitting home alone at my kitchen table, I took several long, deep breaths. When I breathed out, the sharp, tight fear that was gripping my body softened. I buried my head in my hands, and tears again flooded through me. My nervous system, which had been in a heightened fight-or-flight state during the one-hour crisis, slowly began to return to normal. For a long time, I held my hands over my heart and focused on feeling my breath coming in and out of my body.

Fear ebbed and flowed within me while Scott remained in the hospital for the next week. Finally, he was diagnosed with "organizing pneumonia" and came home, very sick and with an oxygen tank.

My family and I were certainly being challenged to hold openness during a fear-filled time. Any illusions we had about our human immortality and invincibility had been erased. Focusing on feeling my breath come in and out of my body during these very difficult moments helped me to not shut down. Choosing to feel each wave of fear as it arose in my body allowed it to move through me and dissipate. Feeling my fear and letting it move through me opens me to the tenderness of being alive. It also created more inner spaciousness for me to experience love and peace, even with the ongoing uncertainty.

The next three exercises have helped many of my clients, and me personally, when fear has taken over. They will help you stay open and let fear move through you during and after stressful experiences.

Breathing through Fear

The next time you are having a stressful experience, breathing through your acute fear and anxiety will help you keep from shutting down in the moment.

First, focus on your breathing. Just breathe in and breathe out for a few moments.

Notice and name the fear or anxiety as it arises in your body. When you name any feeling, including fear, your nervous system automatically starts to calm down.

Next, imagine a warm, golden light flowing down through the top of your head. It flows down into your neck, shoulders, chest, abdomen, hips, and legs before flowing out of your body through your feet.

Continue breathing in and out. Imagine any lingering fear leaving your body, like gray smoke, on every exhale.

Retrain Your Fearful Mind

How do you feel fear in a safe way? The following process, which is a variation of "Retrain Your Negative-Thinking Mind" from chapter 2, interrupts the limbic loop of fear created by our thoughts and feelings.

The next time fear takes over:

1. Become aware. Ask yourself, "What is the fearful thought?"
2. Identify the thought.
3. Come back to your body. Your body is always in the present moment.
4. Take a few minutes to just breathe. Just feel your breath coming in and out of your body. Or you may want to feel the energy pulsing in your hands. When you focus on your breath or the energy pulsing in your hands, your thinking mind stops.
5. Now name the fearful feeling. Use whatever words best reflect the intensity of the fear, such as *worry, anxiety, apprehension,* or *terror.*
6. Where in your body do you feel that feeling? Locate that feeling in your body. Maybe you feel it in your head, your chest, or your stomach area. Maybe you feel it elsewhere.
7. Breathe into the part of your body holding the feeling. Let yourself feel what is there for at least a few minutes.
8. Shift your attention to your lower belly. Put your hand on it and breathe deeply.
9. Come back to the fearful thought you identified in step 2. Replace it with an opposite thought—*I am okay in this moment,* for example.
10. Call to mind a positive memory. Feel the good feelings that arise with that memory. Take those feelings into your body and marinate and savor them.

11. Return to the present moment by focusing again on your breathing. Stay here, in the present moment, with your breath, and enjoy the peace, joy, and other sensations that arise.

Shaking to Release Fear

I share this qigong shaking exercise with clients regularly. It is another way to feel into fear—and any other difficult emotion—and release it.

The next time you are feeling fear, first let yourself feel it in your body.

Now stand with your legs hip width distance apart. Bend your knees gently. Let your arms dangle at your sides.

Start shaking your arms and then your torso.

Imagine any fear or unrest leaving your body as you shake.

Then start shaking your legs and the rest of your body, until you are shaking your entire body.

See your body releasing fear as you keep shaking.

Holding Openness without Being Overwhelmed

My pager went off as I walked out of a patient's room at our local trauma hospital. I was being called down to the emergency room. As I walked into the ER, I heard an announcement: "helicopter ten minutes out." Then I continued into the stabilization room (the STAB room) to find medical staff surrounding a patient who was already there. He had been stabbed. I carefully stepped around the blood on the floor to meet the charge nurse and find out what was going on, who this patient was, and if his family had arrived.

While the medical team was furiously working to locate a laceration in his chest, the nurse and I went to the waiting room, where his family members were pacing the floor. They quickly gathered around us as the nurse told them that the doctors were attending to their loved one. She left the room while I sat with the family, holding space and trying to offer a calming presence. Several family members were crying and talking about their loved one.

My pager went off again. After assuring the family I would return, I went back to the STAB room. It looked like a war zone. There was blood all over the floor, and the patient's chest had been cracked open.

Time ran out. The young man died right in front of all of us.

All the frantic noise and movement in the room suddenly stopped. Everyone stood still and quiet around his gurney. I said a few quiet prayers and a blessing.

The moment ended abruptly as the side doors of the STAB room pushed open. The helicopter whose arrival had been announced when I first arrived in the ER had landed, and a paramedic pilot and crew member were rushing in another patient, a middle-aged man who had been shot. He was not conscious. Another set of medical staff followed the paramedics into another STAB bed area to assess his condition.

One of the doctors who had been working on the young man's stab wounds looked over at me. I had worked with him many times in challenging, dire patient cases. I knew the next steps.

I took a deep breath and focused on feeling the ground underneath my feet as I walked with the doctor to the family waiting area. Silently, I prayed for help and support.

Telling any family that their loved one has died is a gut-wrenching task. As a chaplain, my role was to provide support and comfort. My heart ached with the family of the young man who had just died, and I cried along with them. I spent the next few hours with them, helping pick them up off the floor.

Early on in my career as a trauma chaplain, I'd leave the hospital after shifts like this feeling exhausted and depleted. Even on other, less intense nights, I'd leave feeling off in some way. I also saw many of my colleagues—both chaplains and medical staff—burn out and become brittle from the amount of crises and death we regularly witnessed. If they didn't end up quitting, many of them shut down and became cool and aloof. It quickly became clear to me that I needed to find a way to stay open to what was happening so that I could be helpful to patients and colleagues while not becoming physically, emotionally, and spiritually dysregulated.

I learned how to hold openness safely in these situations by consciously working with my energy field. This subtle electromagnetic field surrounds our human body and typically extends outward about six feet. It comprises physical, emotional, mental, and spiritual energy. This energy field is how we're able to feel and sense the energy around us, including the energy of the environment itself, as well as the other people in it. Sometimes sensing all this surrounding energy is helpful because it allows us to flow with the energy of what's happening and attune to how others are feeling. But if we're not careful, our energy fields can allow us to feel and sense so much that it throws off our own personal energy.

I discovered and fine-tuned some techniques for changing the sensitivity of my energy field so that it could act as a stronger boundary, shielding me from other people's energies and the overall energy of the trauma center. I also learned how to clear other people's energy from my energy field at the end of my shifts. Working intentionally with my energy boundaries allowed me to stay open safely and stay balanced in the intensely stressful situations I encountered daily.

Holding openness means staying open to the flow of life during challenging times. It doesn't mean opening ourselves to negative or overwhelming energies.

Another thing that helped me was regularly taking time to come into the present moment, turn inward, and identify and name whatever feelings were present for me in that moment. Creating some space and being curious about what was happening within was empowering for me and kept me from getting overwhelmed when I was working. I learned how to notice when I was beginning to have a visceral reaction or just starting to feel off. When I realized I was having a strong reaction, I knew I needed to take a break from the situation, if only for a couple of minutes.

Finally, I made a regular habit of grounding myself. Being grounded means we move from our mind into our body. In doing so, we feel supported by the earth and, in my case, by something greater. When we are grounded, we feel our inner strength. We feel supported and rooted. We stay in our power, and nothing, including other people's energy and actions, throws us off-balance. Grounding creates an inner stability that allows us to hold openness and move with the flow of what's happening, even when there is upheaval going on around us.

The first awakening practice has already shown you how to tune in to your inner experience and notice what is present in the moment. The following exercises are some of my favorite techniques for setting and clearing our energy boundaries and for staying grounded.

Setting Energy Boundaries

Setting energy boundaries helps you stay in your power by ensuring that you are not taking in the energy of others, the energy of the news, or the chaotic energy of the world. It doesn't matter whether you are around people in person, talking with people on the phone or on video, or just watching TV. Setting your energy boundaries will help you stay calm and relax your nervous system.

Here are two different methods for setting your energy boundaries. I suggest trying both methods and seeing if one or the other resonates more with you.

Setting your boundaries with visualization: Take a few deep breaths and visualize a bright white force field around you. See it form into a bubble with a hole at the top, above your head. The hole at the top is where love, light, and peace can come in. Visualize this force field extending a good three to five feet around your body. If it feels right, you can also visualize the bubble covered with outward-facing mirrors. Any negative, difficult, or harmful energy that hits this bubble will bounce off and not come into your body or get stuck in the field.

Setting your boundaries with words and intention: Take a few deep breaths. Say out loud or silently, "I now send 70 percent love to everyone and receive 30 percent love in return." You can send love, peace, or any other positive energy you want to send. You can also experiment with the percentages. One day you might send 80 percent love and receive 20 percent back. Another day you can try sending 90 percent love and receiving 10 percent back. Notice how you feel each day and tune in to what percentage feels appropriate for you personally. For me, sending 90 percent love and receiving 10 percent is the perfect ratio that I habitually say every day. These boundaries should help you feel more space, ease, and balance.

If you are in a very tumultuous situation, and the tensions are very high and sharp, you can send love or peace at 100 percent and receive at a 0 percent level. Say out loud or silently, "I now send 100 percent love and receive nothing." Say this several times while you breathe in and out.

I've used this method over many years in a few very challenging situations, and I've found it to be life changing. Sending 100 percent love and receiving nothing allows me to be present and not take in any outside energy. It creates a buffer between me and those around me who are in turmoil. It still helps me today when I'm working with people one-to-one, and I need to be present but not take in any of their energy.

Whichever method you choose, I recommend setting your energy boundaries in the morning before you start your day. At first you can check in and set them again in the middle of the day. Eventually, setting your energy boundaries will become a daily habit, and you'll only need to set them in the morning.

Clearing Your Energy Field

If you've found yourself taking in a lot of energy and being thrown off-balance, this simple exercise will clear your energy field of any energy that is not yours or that you no longer need so that you can feel fully present in your body again.

In a time and place where you will not be interrupted or distracted, say the following statements, filling in each blank with the names or descriptions of the people, places, or situations whose energy you want to clear. Be fully present as you say each statement. As you say them, you can also visualize the connections and attachments as cords that are being cut.

> *I cut all spiritual connections and attachments with _____.*
> *I cut all etheric connections and attachments with _____.*
> *I cut all entity connections and attachments with _____.*
> *I now call back in my full essence and vitality.*

Grounding Exercise

The more centered and grounded you are, the easier it is to hold openness without getting thrown off-balance. I share the following practice with many of my clients to help them come into their body, connect to the earth and universal life force energy, and feel supported and stable.

Stand with your legs hip width distance apart. Let your arms dangle at your side.

Visualized a cord of white light coming down through the top of your head, down your right side, down through your right leg and foot, and into the ground.

See this light travel down into the center of the earth. When it meets the center of the earth, see it release any negative, charged, or heavy emotions you no longer want. Mother Earth will take in and transform these energies.

Next see the white light turn around and make its way back up through the earth toward your body. Along the way, it passes boulders, twigs, and rocks, gathering life-giving energy from the earth as it rises. See it come up through the earth and enter your left foot. See this light travel up your left leg and your left side, bathing and nourishing your body as it travels to the top of your head.

At the top of your head, the light curves back downward and goes back down your right side into the earth again.

Continue visualizing this loop for as long as there is energy you want to release into the earth, always taking in the healing energy of the earth and allowing it to bathe and enliven your body.

Opening to Transformation

Pam's voicemail said she had heard me speak at a local grief consortium group and remembered I had companioned her mother at the end of life seven years before. I instantly remembered her and her mother. Now Pam was requesting to meet with me because her adult son had died by suicide a few months ago.

Over the course of many months, Pam shared her journey of feeling both deep sorrow and deep joy for her son and her life and the many things she had learned along the way. I felt her wide-open heart, her tenderness. I witnessed how she listened deeply within for guidance. She also drew guidance from her connection with nature, all living beings, and God. She told me that her early morning walks in nature filled her soul. She noticed and sensed her son's presence in a wide array of life around her. My heart expanded as I saw and felt her deep openness, her raw emotions, and her ability to be present and take in what was good and life giving.

Pam is more vibrantly alive and aware of the preciousness of life than most people I've encountered.

Amid her grief, which she continues to live through, her curiosity, openness, and wonderment are palpable. Pam is living the questions: What is life teaching me right now? How can I feel into all that life is right now? What does it mean to be alive?

> *[S]uffering is sometimes the sandpaper that awakens people.*
> —Ram Dass, Polishing the Mirror

When we hold openness, we're able to more deeply feel and experience life's sorrows. And that in turn opens us more. We are continually creating space to experience all of life.

Holding openness through loss, grief, and suffering, as well as life's less intense ups and downs, transforms us and moves us into awakening. If we can hold openness in these times, we will transform and feel more fully alive.

Maybe we're grieving the loss of a loved one, the loss of a job, or loss of income. Maybe we're grieving a loss of overall freedom and a sense of ease. Perhaps we're feeling grief in the face of inequity and injustice. Maybe we're feeling grief for all these things and more, all at the same time.

It is easy to withdraw when we are experiencing loss, grief, or suffering. Feeling our emotions and letting them run through us is what allows us to hold openness. Can you start with moments of feeling into your feelings and see how that goes? As you do, can you stay open to any inner knowing and reflections that may surface? Can you take note when you are closed off and notice how that feels? You may even ask yourself the question: How am I closed off today? And ask its opposite: What can give me some life and feed my soul today?

If we can remain open amid difficult times, we can flow with the current of life. We can let it carry us. We can be present with what is happening in the moment and embrace all of life, with all its many edges. We can feel into what sustains us in the moment.

When we hold openness during challenging times, we transform. We feel into the preciousness of being alive. We feel into the range and spectrum of our humanness. We feel into the universal energy that is within and around us. And we awaken.

———————————————

Prayer for Openness

May I follow my breath as I breathe in and out.
May I stay open in the face of my suffering.
May I stay open in the face of my unrest.
May I continue to hold openness.
May I continue to awaken.
May I feel fully alive.

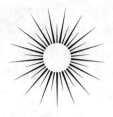

CONCLUSION

Choose to Awaken

LIFE IS SHORT. LIFE IS PRECIOUS.

If you don't awaken to your essence, your aliveness now, but instead wait until it comes when you take your last breath, you miss out on what it means to be alive right now. You miss out on how life can be full, rich, and magical, and you miss the love and guidance that is here for all of us.

Living through the global coronavirus pandemic that began in 2020 has been soul shaping for all of us. It has been a wake-up call, asking each of us what it means to be alive on this earth. Many of us have never had to look directly at death, dying, and the unknown until the pandemic began. And by doing so, we've realized we don't feel fully alive.

There has been great social, political, and economic unrest along with the pandemic. The world is opening and shifting. It's also constantly speeding up, and even with the advancements in technology that have brought us closer together, many people feel isolated and alone. As we are forced to move into a new normal and a new way of being in the world, finding a felt sense of aliveness and deep inner peace is a more urgent need than ever before. Many of us are yearning to feel more whole, grounded, connected, and in touch with life.

Once the soul awakens, the search begins and you can never go back.
—*John O'Donohue,* Anam Cara

I'm inspired by how many people are showing up in my private practice, seeking a feeling of peace, ease, and belonging in their daily lives. It shows me the urgency of this longing to awaken.

I also continue to be amazed by the resiliency of the human spirit. I think our ability to bounce back from pain and suffering and continue growing is our greatest strength as humans. I know that pain, suffering, and other challenges and difficulties can be opportunities for us to keep awakening, if we choose to see them that way.

How might our world change if each of us made the conscious choice to come back to the present moment, connect with something greater, grow our trust, embody love, and hold openness?

How might our world change if each of us really, truly felt fully alive?

I believe more peace would enter into our world. I believe it would be easier for us to accept and love each other. I believe the more conscious and alive each of us becomes, the more peace and ease would have room to flourish between us and ripple out from us.

Living an awakened life out of the center of our soul, we shine our light so that others can find their light.

I know you can find the aliveness, the sparkle, the sense of "oh, so this is what it means to be alive!" if you choose.

Every day is an awakening opportunity.

To be alive is a gift.

All you have to do is say yes.

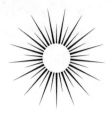

Master List of Exercises

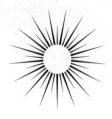

Additional Resources

HERE ARE SOME OF MY FAVORITE, must-read books for going deeper into the five practices and learning more about awakening.

The Most Important Thing: Discovering Truth at the Heart of Life, Adyashanti—an exploration of our ego, the present moment, and what it means to be alive.

Unwinding Anxiety: New Science Shows How to Break the Cycles of Worry and Fear to Heal Your Mind, Judson Brewer, MD, PhD—learn how to identify your triggers and rewire your brain through curiosity, mindfulness, and other practices.

The Spiritual Life, Sri Chinmoy—a short book on life, meaning, and deepening your inner peace.

Soul Lessons and Soul Purpose: A Channeled Guide to Why You Are Here, Sonia Choquette—outlines twenty-two soul lessons that can help us live our purpose.

Start Where You Are: A Guide to Compassionate Living, Pema Chödrön—offers fifty-nine Buddhist principles to help us move through pain, embrace it, and thus become more fully alive.

Energy Healing for Trauma, Stress and Chronic Illness, Cyndi Dale—a powerful guide to help you heal from trauma and chronic health challenges.

Polishing the Mirror: How to Live from Your Spiritual Heart, Ram Dass—a well-known, beloved spiritual teacher explores how we create our life and come into our true nature here and now.

Healing Words: The Power of Prayer and the Practice of Medicine, Larry Dossey, MD—explains how prayer is not only a powerful way to connect with something greater but it can also contribute to our physical healing.

Change Your Thoughts, Change Your Life: Living the Wisdom of the Tao, Wayne W. Dyer—explores eighty-one practices of the Tao Te Ching and how we can apply them into our daily lives.

Breaking the Habit of Being Yourself: How to Lose Your Mind and Create a New One, Dr. Joe Dispenza—how understanding neuroscience, brain chemistry, and biology can help you find inner peace.

The Chemistry of Calm: A Powerful Drug-Free Plan to Quiet Your Fears and Overcome Your Anxiety, Henry Emmons, MD—a holistic approach for healing anxiety and strengthening resilience.

Creative Visualization: Use the Power of Your Imagination to Create What You Want in Your Life, Shakti Gawain—a short read on how we can change our lives through affirmations and imagery.

Neurodharma: New Science, Ancient Wisdom, and Seven Practices of the Highest Happiness, Rick Hanson, PhD—a good reference for Hanson's neuroplasticity model, HEAL.

The Power Is Within You, Louise Hay—a guide to loving and accepting ourselves, moving through fear, accepting change, and living from our heart.

This Thing Called You, Ernest Holmes—a classic book on what it means to live fully.

Healing Ourselves: Biofield Science and the Future of Health, Shamini Jain, PhD—looks at the future of health and healing through an integrative, holistic lens that encompasses both conventional medicine and alternative healing.

Full Catastrophe Living: Using the Wisdom of Your Body and Mind to Face Stress, Pain, and Illness, Jon Kabat-Zinn—a classic book on how we can use various mind-body approaches, including meditation and yoga, to reduce stress and increase health and well-being.

The Power of Purpose: Finding Meaning, Live Longer, Better, Richard J. Leider—how to find your purpose and passion in order to feel alive.

Head to Heart: The 18-inch Journey into Oneself, Master Chunyi Lin—describes how living less from the mind and more from the heart is the path to awakening.

The Upside of Stress: Why Stress Is Good for You, and How to Get Good at It, Kelly McGonigal, PhD—a novel view of stress and a guide for harnessing its helpful benefits.

Dying to Be Me: My Journey from Cancer, to Near Death, to True Healing, Anita Moorjani—Anita has a near-death experience and learns the power of healing and the meaning of life.

How Then, Shall We Live?: Four Simple Questions That Reveal the Beauty and Meaning of Our Lives, Wayne Muller—the first of Miller's four questions is, what do I love? His exploration of this question through prayer, poems, and teachings offers further insights on how to embody love.

Anatomy of the Spirit: The Seven Stages of Power and Healing, Caroline Myss—an introduction to the chakra system described in the Hindu tradition and how to use it for healing and reaching a higher state of consciousness.

Self-Compassion: The Proven Power of Being Kind to Yourself, Kristin Neff, PhD—an introduction to self-compassion, a well-researched, three-part practice that helps support self-love.

Let Your Life Speak: Listening for the Voice of Vocation, Parker Palmer—an important heart-centered book about following your inner voice to find meaning and purpose.

The 5 Second Rule: Transform Your Life, Work, and Confidence with Everyday Courage, Mel Robbins—a great, easy-to-implement way to change your life, break a bad habit, defuse self-doubt and negative self-talk, and rewire your brain.

The Four Agreements: A Practical Guide to Personal Freedom, Don Miguel Ruiz—a classic, short read on how to live your life based on four principles to find happiness and love.

Emotional Clearing: The Handbook of Integrative Processing (1st ed.), John Ruskan—a well-thought-out approach for experiencing, accepting, and releasing our feelings.

The Magic Path of Intuition, Florence Scovel Shinn—how to let go of fear, doubt, and resistance to cultivate intuition and transform your life.

Good Morning, I Love You: Mindfulness and Self-Compassion Practices to Rewire Your Brain for Calm, Clarity, and Joy, Shauna Shapiro, PhD—explores the brain science behind our feelings, citing many studies, and how we can rewire our brain for positivity.

The Untethered Soul: The Journey Beyond Yourself, Michael A. Singer—a dive into self-discovery, present-moment living, and developing our consciousness.

The Power of Now: A Guide to Spiritual Enlightenment, Eckhart Tolle—a must-read for understanding the power of living in the present moment.

A Monk's Guide to Happiness: Meditation in the 21st Century, Gelong Thubten—an easy-to-read book on the power of our mind and how we can create mental stillness, mental space, and happiness.

The Power of Love: Connecting to the Oneness, James Van Praagh—describes how love and acceptance are the keys to opening your heart, connecting with the light within, and connecting with the greater universe.

A Return to Love: Reflections on the Principles of A Course in Miracles, Marianne Williamson—explores the power of choosing love over fear.

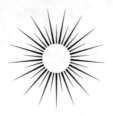

Acknowledgments

I WANT TO THANK Amy Rost, my book coach and developmental editor, who is a true wizard. Your guidance, insight, and spiritual depth are unmatched.

I also want to thank my friends who have walked with me and have been true guides and light: Jac Coverdale, Cyndi Dale, Laurie Edwalds, Ester Gorsky, Heather Heefner, Ellen Hufschmidt, Jack Riordan, and my sister, Nancy Fraser.

Thank you to Dr. Kevin Harrington, for helping me during my soul-shaping years of inner discovery, and to my cherished colleague, gifted healer, and friend Michael Isaacson, for your ongoing guidance.

Thank you, Naren Aryal, at Amplify, for seeing the vision of this book, and Richelle Fredson, for being an invaluable guide on my book-publishing journey.

Thank you to my mom, Carol Owens, who embodies love, deep faith, and prayer—and who has a direct connection to God. And finally, thank you to my mother-in-law, Karen Duncan, who died young but taught me in her death how to live and who opened within me the next steps on my journey.

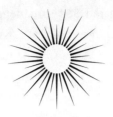

About the Author

CATHERINE DUNCAN, MA, BCC, is passionate about whole-person healing. Her focus as an integrative spiritual consultant is emotional and spiritual health. With a reverence for the sacredness of life, she companions individuals who are struggling with chronic illness, life transitions, grief and loss, and those searching for more meaning and purpose.

She sees clients through her own private practice, Learning to Live, LLC, and as a consultant with Minnesota Personalized Medicine, an integrative medical practice in Minneapolis.

In her work, she draws on her experience as a board-certified chaplain and certified spiritual director; her training in positive neuroplasticity with Rick Hanson, PhD; and her education in a range of alternative healing modalities, including Reiki, Healing Touch, qigong, the Emotional Freedom Technique (EFT)/tapping, and sound healing.

As a public speaker, she frequently delivers talks on stress and resiliency, self-compassion, self-care, neuroplasticity, and awakening to organizations and companies in person and virtually. Her writing is featured on the website for the University of Minnesota's Earl E. Bakken Center for Spirituality and Healing, the Institute for Well-Being in Law's website, and in the textbook *Integrative Medicine* by David Rakel, MD (5th edition, Elsevier, November 2022).

Catherine has served as a spiritual-care provider with Fairview Home Care and Hospice, Hennepin Healthcare, and the Good Samaritan Society. An ordained minister with the United Church of Christ, she received her MA in theology and her spiritual direction certificate from St. Catherine University (St. Paul, Minnesota). She also holds a master of divinity equivalency from United Theological Seminary (New Brighton, Minnesota).

In addition to her deep professional background, Catherine teaches from her three personal awakening experiences, including a brush with death that opened her gifts as a mystic and intuitive. These spiritual gifts, which include the ability to see spirits, support her work of helping people open into their souls.

She lives in Minneapolis with her husband and two dogs, Bella and Gigi, and is the mother of two adult children. For more, please visit her website: learningtolive.org.